Abuse
of the Doctor–Patient
Relationship

Abuse
of the Doctor–Patient
Relationship

Edited by Fiona Subotsky,
Susan Bewley and Michael Crowe

RCPsych Publications

RCPsych Publications is an imprint of the Royal College of Psychiatrists,
17 Belgrave Square, London SW1X 8PG
http://www.rcpsych.ac.uk

British Library Cataloguing-in-Publication Data.
A catalogue record for this book is available from the British Library.

ISBN 978-1-904671-37-4

Distributed in North America by Publishers Storage and Shipping Company.

The views presented in this book do not necessarily reflect those of the Royal College of
Psychiatrists, and the publishers are not responsible for any error of omission or fact.

Printed by Bell & Bain Limited, Glasgow, UK.

Contents

Figures, tables and boxes

Figures

Tables

Boxes

Contributors

Susan Bewley Consultant Obstetrician, King's Health Partners Women's Services, St Thomas' Hospital, London

Dinesh Bhugra President, Royal College of Psychiatrists, and Professor of Mental Health and Cultural Diversity, Institute of Psychiatry, King's College London, London

Peter Carter Chief Executive, Royal College of Nursing, London

Ngozi Chukwudi Medical Student, King's College London, London

Michael Crowe Psychiatrist in private practice, previously Consultant Psychiatrist, South London and Maudsley NHS Trust, Honorary Senior Lecturer, Institute of Psychiatry, King's College London, London

Patricia Crowley Associate Professor of Obstetrics and Gynaecology, Trinity College, Dublin, and Consultant Obstetrician and Gynaecologist, Coombe Women's and Infants' University Hospital, Dublin

Chess Denman Consultant Psychiatrist in Psychotherapy, Fulbourn Hospital, Cambridge

Dawn Devereux Director of Public Support, The Clinic for Boundary Studies, London, and psychotherapist in private practice

Bobbie Farsides Professor of Clinical and Biomedical Ethics, Brighton and Sussex Medical School, Brighton

Tanya Garrett Clinical and Forensic Psychologist, Honorary Senior Lecturer, University of Birmingham, Birmingham

Peter Haughton Senior Adviser in Medical Ethics and Law, School of Medicine, King's College London, London

David Misselbrook General Practitioner, Lewisham; Dean, Royal Society of Medicine, London

Andrew Pickering Medicolegal Adviser, Medical Protection Society, Leeds

Pete Snowden   Medical Director, Calverton Hill Hospital, Partnerships in Care, Arnold, Nottinghamshire

Claire Spake   Medical Student, King's College London, London

Julie Stone   Independent Consultant in Healthcare Law and Ethics; Visiting Professor in Ethics, Peninsula Medical School, Exeter

Fiona Subotsky   Emeritus Consultant Child and Adolescent Psychiatrist, South London and Maudsley NHS Trust; Honorary Archivist, Royal College of Psychiatrists, London

Joan Trowell   Emeritus Fellow, Nuffield Department of Medicine, University of Oxford, previously GMC Council member and Chairman of the GMC Fitness to Practise Committee

Foreword

The doctor–patient relationship is at the core of treatment, whether psychological, pharmacological or surgical. There is considerable evidence that even when treatment involves no more than a prescription, the expectations and the nature of the therapeutic encounter dictate the response and acceptance of treatment. The doctor–patient interaction works at various levels and both sides respond to this, depending upon their experience, education, gender, ethnicity, age and other factors. The nature of the therapeutic interaction in psychiatry – in risk assessment and psychotherapy sessions especially – ensures that the psychiatrist is in a powerful position. This may lead to physical, sexual or emotional exploitation of the vulnerable individual, sometimes unintentionally but at other times deliberately.

Ethical issues related to such encounters are at the heart of this volume, which deals with the context, prevalence and sequelae of such events, and also considers prevention. Healthcare professionals have their own personality characteristics and life experiences, as do patients, which should not interfere with therapy but sometimes may. The editors are to be congratulated for providing a pragmatic and extremely helpful overview. They show that to improve upon the present situation there needs to be an increase in awareness and education, alongside better monitoring and regulation.

This book should be essential reading not only for trainees and psychiatrists, but also for other health professionals. The therapeutic encounter must be safe and beneficial for the patient. Both vulnerable patients and their carers must have full confidence in the probity and ethical values of a treating psychiatrist and the medical profession as a whole. It is up to the profession to set the standards and ensure that these are met. This book provides a welcome first step for raising standards. I hope it will be read widely.

Dinesh Bhugra
President
Royal College of Psychiatrists

Introduction: mapping the territory

Fiona Subotsky, Susan Bewley and Michael Crowe

The breaking of boundaries in doctor–patient relationships has been discussed in many recent publications, mainly from North America, Australia and New Zealand, where there have also been extensive modifications to codes of medical practice as a result (see Sarkar, 2004). In view of the lessons learned from recent scandals, it is timely to write about the British experience, especially as the delivery of healthcare, the legal and financial contexts, and even the favoured theoretical understandings are so different. In this book, we have concentrated on the paradigm case of the breaching of sexual boundaries, although other areas of transgression are also discussed. The greatest risk appears to exist in the specialties of psychiatry, gynaecology and general practice, and so it is appropriate that this educational book has a multidisciplinary authorship and editorship.

The genesis of the book was in the Royal College of Psychiatrists' need to respond to both the process and the recommendations of the Kerr/Haslam Inquiry. This formal inquiry, chaired by Nigel Pleming QC, examined how, despite complaints of sexual abuse by patients over many years, two male psychiatrists working from the same hospital in the north of England were able to continue professionally without challenge (Department of Health, 2005; Kennedy, 2006). By reflecting on these events and other cases of boundary transgression, we hope readers may help avoid the repetition of such occurrences.

Are we perhaps too optimistic that people are interested in the topic of abuse within the doctor–patient relationship? After all, the public response to the final report of the Kerr/Haslam Inquiry was very muted. On the other hand, heightened interest in particularly shocking cases seems only to raise denial or distancing from the profession, and demands for extreme punishment and increased regulation from others. Between these two extremes doctors must recognise that it is by being aware of the need for professional boundaries that the vital trust of the public may be maintained. Thus, the Royal College of Physicians' report (2005) *Doctors in Society: Medical Professionalism in a Changing World* defines professionalism as: 'a set of values, behaviours and relationships that underpins the trust the public has in doctors'.

Unequal relationships

Abuses, and taboos to prevent them, do not occur in medicine alone. Any unequal relationship has the potential for sexual abuse and abuse of power built into it. Priests and parishioners, teachers and pupils, sports coaches and their trainees, producers and actors, and above all parents and their children should be in relationships in which sex is expected not to occur. This is for the very good reason that the less powerful member of the dyad is at a disadvantage in terms of influence, and often age, and therefore not able to give free, informed and voluntary consent to what is happening. The trusting relationship puts the more senior member in a position resembling a parent: *in loco parentis* is generally used to characterise the teacher–pupil relationship, but could equally be used to describe the doctor–patient or priest–parishioner relationship, without carrying the negative associations of paternalism. It is perhaps significant at the present time, when authority is being challenged as never before, that there is an outcry about sexual abuse by priests, about incest within families, about sexual harassment within military training academies and about sexual abuse within therapeutic relationships of all sorts, including medical, psychological and psychotherapeutic.

The purpose of rules

The enforcement of boundaries within unequal relationships is based on good reasoning. Despite fashionable movements to turn the doctor–patient relationship into a partnership of equals, this can never be achieved. Doctors and therapists must be constrained by legal and ethical duties of confidentiality, consent and competence in ways which are not necessary for patients. Trust is required for patients to tell secrets, to take potentially harmful medications and to undergo operations when unconscious. The construction, maintenance and repair of professional boundaries is a one-sided responsibility. Medical professionalism itself is threatened not only by the few doctors who infringe appallingly but also by the many whose infringements appear trivial at first.

There are many stages on the slippery slope towards the breach of a boundary within a therapeutic relationship. These can include the giving and receiving of gifts, the sharing of personal information by the doctor/ therapist, socialising with the client/patient, entering into commercial transactions outside those involved in therapy itself, the disclosing by the doctor/therapist of personal information or problems, and eventually by the breaking of the greatest taboo, that of sexual touching. Sometimes these initial infringements are part of a grooming process by a therapist wanting to progress to an intimate relationship with a client, but at other times they are made innocently and with good intention. However, once boundaries are breached it then becomes more difficult to restore a therapeutic relationship in which the proper boundaries are respected.

A multidisciplinary matter

Our brief, as shown by the range of contributions, is one that embraces different medical specialties, and other areas where counselling, psychotherapy and similar activities take place. There is a particular risk in the fields of counselling and psychotherapy, where therapist (or counsellor) and client may be in regular one-to-one contact for a prolonged period, and the patient may be both more vulnerable psychologically and less likely to be believed. However, what applies to mental health practitioners is also true to a lesser extent for the majority of doctors, especially those who see patients regularly, perform intimate examinations, or have knowledge of their patients' lives that their patients would prefer to be kept secret.

Ethics and harm

Of foremost importance are ethical principles, discussed by a number of contributors, but particularly in Chapter 1 by Bobbie Farsides, a medical ethicist who reflects on John Stuart Mill's injunction against harm. She emphasises the obligation placed on the therapist to work within defined boundaries and ensure that the encounter is therapeutic, despite the seeming intimacy of the situation. The harmfulness of boundary violation may be difficult to research quantitatively, but attending to the patient's voice has rightly become part of mainstream medical evaluation and education, and so Dawn Devereux's contribution, 'The patient's perspective', follows (Chapter 2). She writes from the point of view of a psychodynamically trained non-medical psychotherapist who has developed expertise in treating patients who have been previously abused by therapists and has also researched published accounts of such treatment experiences. She draws attention to the phenomenon of 'bystanding' – the wider culpability of those who witness or know but do nothing – perhaps a widespread experience in health services.

Witnessing, observing and reflecting are what Peter Haughton's medical students are asked to do in their course on ethics at King's College Medical School. With two medical student co-authors, Haughton presents ideas and problems regarding medical education that have arisen in the course (Chapter 3). He thus provides some theoretical background and reflection on real examples of poor practice and the dilemmas of how to respond.

Context

The past may reveal patterns that are less clear to us when close up. So a brief historical approach follows, looking first at the development of Western medical codes of ethics and early British regulation through the

General Medical Council (GMC) and then at some particular cases of egregious boundary breaking, and how they were responded to at the time (Chapter 4). The difficulties of discovering the prevalence of even clear-cut boundary breaking are reviewed by Tanya Garrett, a clinical psychologist with a long-standing interest in this area (Chapter 5). The statistics about present rates of abuse largely relate to psychiatry and surely are underestimates, as they are mostly based on self-reports. Nevertheless, what is known, primarily from studies in the USA, Canada, Australia and New Zealand, gives considerable cause for concern, while data from the UK are extremely limited.

In response to the Kerr/Haslam Inquiry, guidance and professional recommendations were developed by the Royal College of Psychiatrists (RCPsych), the institution which has most of the UK's consultant psychiatrists as members, and is responsible for education and standard setting in psychiatry. Fiona Subotsky, who was the College officer responsible for liaising with the Inquiry, outlines this process as it developed (Chapter 6) – a process which needs to continue as greater understanding emerges of the abuse of mental health patients by professionals. Indeed, the production of this book is a further attempt to increase awareness and help prevention.

Specialties

David Misselbrook, a practising general practitioner and current Dean of the Royal Society of Medicine, looks at the culture of general practice in the UK, with its pressures of time and demand (Chapter 7). These produce tensions between ideals of good practice and practicality, which are often a cause of professional stress. He outlines formal theoretical attacks on the medical power structure, from Foucault, Illich and Kennedy, and illustrates the abuse of medical power with several examples. While expressing hope that measures such as audit and revalidation may help, he thinks complete success is unlikely.

The violation of sexual boundaries has been examined in detail especially by psychoanalytically trained and practising psychiatrists. Chess Denman is a consultant psychiatrist in psychotherapy who looks at boundary violations in psychotherapy (Chapter 8). She explains related psychodynamic ideas such as the role of dependent attachment in the patient and unconscious sadistic motivation in the therapist. These phenomena occur in the processes of transference and countertransference, but are not confined to psychodynamic treatments. The field of sexual therapy, reviewed by Michael Crowe (Chapter 9), might be assumed to be a particularly high-risk area. In consequence, one association has developed a strong and explicit professional code in the UK, which includes the need for supervision and for chaperones.

Obstetrics and gynaecology are areas of medical practice which necessitate genital examination of an exclusively female clientele. Patricia Crowley,

Associate Professor of Obstetrics and Gynaecology in Dublin, advises on the prevention of abuse by the appropriate use of chaperones, better information for patients about what to expect and better education for doctors, nurses and midwives (Chapter 10). She warns that the dynamics of the doctor–patient relationship can easily lead to excessive intervention, whether through the doctor's vested interest or desire to progress modern techniques, or the wish of the patient for ready solutions. Ideally, these specialties should be a force for the improvement of women's rights in health.

Peter Carter, Chief Executive of the Royal College of Nursing, considers the range of possible reasons for abuse by nurses, from the cultural and systemic to the intrapersonal (Chapter 11). He presents the case of David Britten – a senior nurse who sexually abused many young women patients in an eating disorders ward – and has some illustrative accounts from nurses who have admitted abuse. By way of contrast, a model example of good practice in the management of a case of alleged assault is given; it shows what persistence and dedication are necessary to secure a just result.

Prevention

Many of the contributors make recommendations on the prevention of boundary abuse, but evidence of success is difficult to obtain, as the baseline is so poorly defined and monitored. Fortunately, this situation is beginning to be improved in the UK, through the work of the National Patient Safety Agency and the National Clinical Assessment Service. Primary prevention may be considered to include clarification of principles, education for doctors and information for patients. Secondary prevention is generally understood as aiming at identifying risk areas and ensuring early identification of problems in order to react appropriately. This organisational level is targeted in Chapter 12, 'Medical management', by Fiona Subotsky, which advises a systematic approach to policies and audit to help prevent abuse, as formal inquiries have always shown up great weaknesses in these areas.

At the tertiary level of prevention (damage limitation), abuse has occurred and the abusive (or possibly abusive) doctor has to be dealt with. Peter Snowden, a forensic psychiatrist and medical director, writes about the range of sanctions and remediation available in the UK (Chapter 13). In terms of the latter, there is little systematic provision, unfortunately. While there is greater provision in the USA, it is still not yet clear what is effective enough to guarantee patient safety.

As in other areas of medicine, there can be false positives and false negatives. The medical defence organisations see another side of the picture and can also offer much useful advice to doctors. Andrew Pickering, a medico-legal adviser, notes that doctors are subject to 'multiple jeopardy', as complaints may be formally raised and action taken against them in a number of different forums (Chapter 14). The accused doctors may be hampered from defending themselves by the restrictions of confidentiality, but their livelihoods are threatened irrespective of the truth or otherwise of allegations.

Regulation of medical and other health practitioners has been debated at length in the past decade, and we are fortunate to have a contribution by Julie Stone (Chapter 15), who led the Council for Healthcare Regulatory Excellence's project 'Clear Sexual Boundaries' (www.chre.org.uk) which produced so much useful material on the topic (see Appendix 3). She argues that while the CHRE has a major role to play in promoting professional excellence for patient safety, government support will nonetheless be critical for success.

The primary medical regulator in the UK is the GMC, whose practice and advice have recently been shaped by major scandals of errant doctors and the consequent inquiries and recommendations. The chapter by Joan Trowell, a past medical member of the GMC Council, outlines much of the GMC's current procedures and guidance in relation to boundary issues (Chapter 16). Real case examples from the GMC are included in Appendix 4.

Major themes

Case studies are provided in most of the chapters and also in the Appendices. This is partly because of their intrinsic interest and educational value, but also because the abstract metaphor 'boundary violation' conceals within it a huge range of behaviour, including the truly shocking and near unspeakable. It is this 'not speaking' which has contributed to so much abuse being permitted to continue for so long.

Professional self-interest, the abuse of power, risks and the rights of vulnerable patients, especially women and people who are mentally ill, have all been considered in this book. While there may be indignation, there is no cause for despair, as much could be improved. We hope that this book will speak to readers so that more doctors, therapists, nurses, trainees and students will reflect on boundaries and work on their maintenance.

References

Department of Health (2005) *The Kerr/Haslam Inquiry*. TSO (The Stationery Office).

Kennedy, P. (2006) Kerr/Haslam Inquiry into sexual abuse of patients by psychiatrists. *Psychiatric Bulletin*, **30**, 204–206.

Royal College of Physicians (2005) *Doctors in Society: Medical Professionalism in a Changing World*. Report of a Working Party (J. Cumberlege, chair) of the Royal College of Physicians of London. RCP.

Sarkar, S. P. (2004) Boundary violation and sexual exploitation in psychiatry and psychotherapy: a review. *Advances in Psychiatric Treatment*, **10**, 312–320.

CHAPTER 1

The ethical importance of boundaries to intimacy

Bobbie Farsides

Overview

Therapists occupy a privileged space in their clients' lives and have a relationship that falls between the public and the private domain in a challenging way. An ethical responsibility therefore exists for the individual therapist to ensure that his or her relationship with a client remains clearly wedded to its therapeutic purpose. This obligation must be recognised at the outset of the therapeutic encounter and will define the boundaries within which any work must be conducted. Even though the work to be done will entail an intimacy more common to private encounters, the relationship must be conducted with a propriety judged appropriate and fitting by professional peers. Setting boundaries is both a professional and an individual duty, the fulfilment of which protects both therapist and client.

Introduction

Sometimes you accept an invitation with a mixture of enthusiasm and trepidation, as was the case when I was approached to contribute to this volume. Just as you might relish a dinner party invitation when you know and like the other guests and feel that you have some interesting stories to tell, so as an academic I relish joining with others to explore a shared interest, particularly when my expertise is recognised and acknowledged. It is much more daunting to go to a dinner party when you know only the hostess, and the other guests come from her world rather than yours. Similarly, it is challenging to address the readers of this book, an expert audience, on a topic about which they have medical knowledge and expertise I do not share. As in the dinner party analogy, I can only hope to come up with some good stories to share, and a level of common understanding that will help the evening go well.

On this occasion, my perspective is that of an ethicist with a particular interest in the experience of healthcare professionals who operate in morally complex areas (Alderson *et al*, 2002; Ehrich *et al*, 2007). My work is also informed by my earlier academic career in which I studied and taught political philosophy, and by my personal experience as a woman growing up riding the second wave of British feminism. I have not experienced the type of therapeutic relationship upon which I will reflect, and ask for understanding of my necessarily lay perspective. It is for readers to judge what happens when they fill in the gaps with their own experiences, as therapist or client.

The therapeutic relationship

Relationships between consenting adults have generally been deemed a core component of our private lives. As such, in a liberal democratic society, they remain largely outside the reach of the state and its laws. Certain relationships become formalised and legitimised through the intervention of courts and registrars, but the way in which those relationships are subsequently conducted remains profoundly private. This means that, for some, the private realm is a safe space in which they can explore their individuality and develop their relationships with significant others. But for others, the private realm is a threatening or positively destructive environment in which their personal safety and well-being can be threatened. A constant challenge for those charged with the protection of others is to find a way to respect the private lives of others while at the same time ensuring that bad things are not happening behind closed doors.

The second-wave feminists, of the late 1960s and 1970s, who campaigned famously under the banner of 'the personal is political', understood this dilemma well (Nicholson, 1997). Their agenda was, in large part, driven by a concern for the invisibility of sexual discrimination, the abuse of women within the home, and the systematic exclusion of women from the public sphere. These feminists appealed to, rather than rejected, liberal doctrine by locating harms within the private sphere and then stating that they should nonetheless be the law's business. In taking this approach, they both challenged and absorbed the idea that the most justifiable reason for intervening in the private lives of citizens is the need to prevent harm to others. Where harms were universally experienced by women, and indirectly sanctioned by the state, the issue became political in the traditional sense of the term, despite the experience of those harms being seen as profoundly personal, situated in the home rather than in the public arena.

In terms of public and private, the relationship between therapist and client is an interesting hybrid. The client leaves his or her home and enters the therapist's professional space. This may be in a clearly designated public place such as a hospital or other institution, or may be an intimate quasi-private space within the therapist's home. Wherever the space exists, it may give clues to the therapist's personal taste and interests, or it may be an utterly impersonal space, available as a work-space to others at different times.

In anything other than the most acute setting, one imagines that the ambience within the space will be carefully constructed in the interests of encouraging openness and trust, and much work will be done to make the client comfortable. The client brings problems to the therapist which may be more or less invisible to the outside world. The close and often intense one-to-one encounter that occurs in this space will be more reminiscent of encounters within the private spaces of the client's life than those experienced in public spaces. Conversations will be deep and revealing, confidences will be shared, and by assisting the client in dealing with problems the therapist will necessarily have to learn much more about the person who is their patient than, say, the orthopaedic surgeon or ophthalmologist.

It is possible, at least, that a closeness will develop that mimics and, in some senses, transcends that achieved with any of the client's significant others. Some of the information shared could be unpalatable for the therapist to hear, as difficult subjects will arise, but similarly the information revealed and examined could elicit feelings of empathy, admiration or attraction, which in other circumstances could be the type of response that would move a relationship on to another level.

It is therefore crucial for therapists to expertly construct the therapeutic relationship and manage the encounters that occur in the therapeutic space. One step towards this would be to ensure appropriate boundaries around their own feelings and responses, feeding them positively into the therapeutic project rather than allowing them to become part of a developing private relationship between two necessarily intimate individuals. This project needs to begin *long before* there is any question of impropriety as defined by law or professional guidance. A therapist in training must acknowledge the need to develop his or her skills in constructing and maintaining appropriate boundaries in relationships with clients. And those charged with training therapists must work to ensure that their students will be equipped with the skills required to do so.

It seems clear that a first step in constructing a healthy therapeutic relationship is an acknowledgement of the fact that the relationship is purpose-driven; thus, any feelings or actions played out within the relationship must serve that purpose. Similarly, the nature of the relationship must be fit for purpose. An interesting question then arises regarding whether, or to what extent, it might be appropriate to allow a potentially 'dangerous' intimacy to develop in the interest of achieving therapeutic goals. In a sense, the question being asked is whether boundaries are fixed and non-negotiable and recognisably the same across all cases, or whether there is room for experimentation in the interests of therapeutic advantage.

The need for professionalism

Clearly, the nature of this type of therapeutic relationship lends itself to a complex blurring of the private and the public, in terms of the space in which it occurs, the conversations shared and the potential responses and reactions of therapist and client. This being the case, there is the potential for relationships to head off in radically different directions if both parties simply allow themselves to go where the experience takes them. One way to manage the issue is to incorporate the notion of professionalism explicitly within the relationship and thereby ensure that one party is constrained in terms of what he or she can, and will, allow to happen.

A healthy professional–client relationship relies on the prior recognition of boundaries; hence the old adage of 'not mixing business and pleasure' arises, because the boundaries cannot be adequately set if a different type of relationship pre-exists the contractual exchange. A persistent trial of everyday life entails conducting relationships with those from whom one purchases services in a manner that demonstrates appropriate respect and concern, without losing the possibility of making appropriate demands or expressing dissatisfaction at the service provided. This problem of etiquette may not be present in the therapist–client relationship but other problems can arise. Part of the therapist's duty rests with acknowledging the possibility and preparing for it.

In the therapist–client relationship some boundaries are conventionally well recognised, such as the importance of regularity and timekeeping – the containment of encounters within specific time and space. Unlike the supportive friend or long-suffering spouse, the therapist allows the client into a designated space for a carefully negotiated amount of time. Therapists can therefore place clear limits on their availability in ways that those in the personal sphere cannot. Conversations can be interrupted and important issues carried over to a future session. This provides a useful reminder of the different nature of the therapeutic relationship, despite the fact that, during the time shared, it may seem very similar to relationships the client values and relies upon in private life.

The professional will have explicit duties of care to the client which are legally and professionally enforceable, such as the duty of confidentiality. This will be a comfort to the client, who may otherwise fear the seepage of information into the private domain. However, it is important to recognise that it is a *professional* as opposed to personal obligation which must be negotiated (as opposed to assumed). Experienced therapists will make it clear what can and cannot remain confidential, and as professionals they will have access to guidance and support on this issue. They will exercise a degree of discretion possibly uncommon among friends and family. They will (ideally) be far apart from their client's social circles, but will also be responsible for judging the danger attaching to truths shared, and they will at times have a clear responsibility to act upon information received.

The therapist will also work hard to retain the nature of the relationship as clearly and unambiguously therapeutic, in the face of any potential shifts in its nature. In some respects, this is part and parcel of the therapeutic process. For example, the therapist must recognise the possibility of transference; but it is also important that she or he recognises the possibility of less therapeutically explicable shifts, and constantly questions whether the relationship remains consistent with the therapeutic purpose.

In dry terms, being a professional entails membership of a professional group or body governed by shared standards of probity and (hopefully) good sense. Being a good professional also means that one should be open to the idea of self-regulation in the absence of clear guidance or explicit standards. In its richest sense, one's status as a professional is another interesting hybrid. Whatever your professional role you cannot lose your personal, private self completely, yet you must allow yourself to be supervised and potentially restricted from acting in ways which run counter to your professional duties. As a private individual you might experience this as challenging, unnecessary or maybe even damaging. Mindful professionals should be subject to an ongoing internal dialogue that helps to pull their personal self in line with their professional duties and role, but also allows their personal self to step away when that is not possible.

Building trust, negotiating relationships

In the public realm, professionalism is in large part about setting standards of good practice, disseminating them effectively to relevant parties and applying sanctions to those who do not meet those standards. Sometimes, however, the standards within a professional group slip or fail to adjust to broader societal shifts. The work of modern bioethics has been, in part, to shift modern medical culture towards a more explicit recognition of the need for sound ethical governance (Jonsen, 1993). There has been an explicit need to move on from the abuses of the past, such as enforced sterilisation of those with a mental impairment, retention of human body parts and conscription into medical research (see Chapter 4 regarding historical abuses).

Initially, bioethics borrowed heavily from the social contract theory of political philosophers. Doctors as professionals have similarly invoked the contractual model at a macro- and micro-level, with international medical associations signing charters and declarations, and individual doctors operating explicitly and implicitly within contracts of care which distribute rights and responsibilities between the healthcare professional and the client.

In recent times, bioethics discourse has also acknowledged the limitations of the legalistically characterised contractual model and has re-incorporated familiar concepts from traditional medical discourse, such as trust, the promotion of best interests and the idea of authorisation. This is not to rule out the possibility or importance of explicit consent in particular cases, but rather it allows for a further discussion of the moral landscape where consent is problematic or absent. The relationship between a therapist and client seems particularly suited to a combination of 'regulatory' mechanisms, some explicitly contractual, others coming out of the underlying trust and mutual respect inherent in a well-constructed and well-managed relationship.

As previously observed, the relationship between the therapist and client will sometimes look little different from that between the client as a private individual and those who care about, and for, him or her in private life. Yet we understand that there is a need for boundaries to be in place because the therapist–client relationship is a variant of the doctor–patient relationship, which is *not* an element of an individual's private life. The therapist conducts the relationship in his or her role as a professional, which is a role defined and regulated in the public sphere. The client 'buys' the professional's services either directly or indirectly in a publicly regulated marketplace.

The space in which the relationship is conducted is relevant, not only because it makes it subject to the law, as it is outside the protected private sphere, but also because it makes the individual relationship subject to the structural features of the context within which it occurs. This is specifically relevant in the healthcare setting, where complex power structures exist which, in turn, help to define the relationship between the doctor and patient, the well and unwell, the client and therapist.

Power and harm

At the beginning, I introduced the notion of the public–private divide in order then to explore the ambiguity of the therapist–client relationship in terms of this dichotomy. What remains clear, however, is that the therapeutic purpose of the relationship and its existence in the public sphere mean that it should be managed and regulated, both directly by the individual therapist and indirectly by the relevant professional body. The moral justification for this lies in the need to prevent harm to either the client or the therapist.

The 'harm principle' is a key component of John Stuart Mill's account of liberty. In describing the 'appropriate region of human liberty' he famously stated that, as well as freedom of conscience, expression and association, 'the principle requires liberty of tastes and pursuits; of framing the plan of our life to suit our own character; of doing as we like, subject to such consequences as may follow; without impediment from our fellow-creatures, *so long as what we do does not harm them even though they should think our conduct foolish, perverse, or wrong*' (Mill, 1859; emphasis added).

Herein lies the idea at the core of the principle of autonomy, which has become so central to Anglo-American bioethics. While autonomy and liberty need to be distinguished from one another (and the role of autonomy should not be overplayed), it is nonetheless important to acknowledge that, within liberal society, individuals have the right to govern their own lives in line with their values and beliefs, and that they may do so even if their actions are 'foolish, perverse, or wrong'. The limitation on this right comes from the corresponding duty thereby not to harm, or unreasonably impede, the autonomy of other individuals.

It is an empirical question whether a relationship between a particular therapist and a particular patient which breaks out of professionally defined and wisely acknowledged boundaries will lead to either party being harmed. It is too easy a step to define all clients as vulnerable and all therapists as powerful and then conclude that any relationship between the two is necessarily dysfunctional and potentially abusive unless it is clearly situated inside professional boundaries. However, it is also true that the boundaries are integral to the therapeutic process, and the key relationship between a therapist and client must remain just that – a professional and caring relationship between an individual with an expressed need and another individual with the expertise to address it. Just as we feel able to bare our bodies to a doctor because we feel confident to assume that he or she will have been trained to see it in a functional, non-judgemental and non-sexual way, so we must feel able to open our hearts and minds to a therapist expecting the same, essentially forensic, response.

If therapists allow a connection with a particular patient to go beyond the purely professional, they must question not only their ability to treat that particular person but also their more generalised professional duty to prioritise the best interest of the patient and avoid doing harm. To move outside their professional expertise into a private relationship is to embark on something inevitably uncertain and potentially dangerous.

Conclusion

A therapeutic relationship is built upon the needs of one party and the expertise of another. In practising his or her art, the therapist will inevitably enter the client's private realm of thought, and the intimacy this creates will sometimes lead one or both parties to desire further intimacy and a shift in the status of the relationship. In order to remain true to the initial purpose of the relationship, this cannot be permitted. This being so, it is important from the outset for the therapist to construct a boundaried notion of intimacy which is robust and fit for purpose. In doing so, the therapist creates a safe space in which much can be shared and within which the therapeutic project can advance. If the client tries to move the relationship to another place, the therapist must resist. Similarly, if the therapist feels drawn to the client in anything other than a properly professional manner, the therapist must resist. The therapeutic project can continue only for as long as the appropriate boundaries stay in place.

References

Alderson, P., Farsides, B. & Williams, C. (2002) Examining ethics in practice: health service professionals' evaluations of in-hospital ethics seminars. *Nursing Ethics*, **9**, 508–521.

Ehrich, K., Williams, C., Farsides, B., *et al* (2007) Choosing embryos: ethical complexity in staff accounts of PGD. *Sociology of Health and Illness*, **29**, 1091–1106.

Jonsen, A. R. (ed.) (1993) 'The Birth of Bioethics'. *Hastings Center Report*, **23**, no. 6 (special supplement).

Mill, J. S. (1859) *On Liberty* (ed. J. Robson), Collected Works, xviii, 225–226 [i, 12]. Routledge, 1996.

Nicholson, L. J. (1997) *The Second Wave: A Reader in Feminist Theory*. Routledge.

CHAPTER 2

The patient's perspective: impact and treatment

Dawn Devereux

Overview

Knowledge of the patient's perspective on the impact of sexual abuse by health-care professionals has been enhanced in recent years by the publication of numerous first-person accounts of professional abuse. The aim of this chapter is to integrate patient and professional perspectives in order to elucidate aspects of sexual abuse that are underrepresented in the literature. The emphasis here is on prevention, and particular attention is paid to those factors that patients identify as important in the development of an abusive relationship. The consequences of the experience of abuse are discussed in terms of the complex nature of subsequent treatment needs. Also considered is the effect that a protracted complaints process may have on treatment and recovery.

Introduction

It should be made clear at the outset that the phrase 'sexual abuse' is used in this chapter in its broadest sense, to include anything sexual within a therapeutic relationship, from flirtatious behaviour (Box 2.1) to rape. Experts in the field now emphasise that sexual abuse should not be considered in a simplistic linear manner, particularly in terms of its effect on the patient (Gabbard & Lester, 1995). As a result, there is growing recognition that any form of sexualised or exploitative behaviour within the consulting room can have profound and devastating consequences.

Self-authored accounts of exploitative experiences of psychotherapy began in 1976 with Julie Roy's book *Betrayal* (Freeman & Roy, 1976) followed by Ellen Plasil's (1985) *Therapist* and Carolyn Bates' and Annette Brodsky's (1988) *Sex in the Therapy Hour*. Such accounts have proliferated during the past three decades, such that there is now an extensive patient-authored literature on all forms of sexual exploitation in psychotherapy. In research terms, this literature is an important naturally occurring data source, as

---

Box 2.1 'I felt powerless'

The following extract is from *Surviving Complaints Against Counsellors and Psychotherapists* (Casemore, 2001, p. 2).

During this time he brought up the subject of sex. He spoke at length on the subject, in a kind of caressing and gentle tone. The atmosphere in the room seemed to me to be electric, and yet as always, I told myself that it was probably part of the therapy, and any other interpretation was possibly just my imagination.

On one occasion he pointed out that as we were born in the same year and had particular stars, it was meant to mean that we were very compatible, especially as we were opposite sexes. Never having believed in any such nonsense myself I found I was feeling delighted by this revelation and sure now that he was trying to tell me something. Another time I asked him if he ever had clients who scared him when working alone in the building. He looked at me hard, paused for several seconds and then pointed his finger at me almost accusingly and said 'you are the client who scares me'. I knew then what he meant and yet I felt powerless to do or say anything very much in response. I just kind of laughed it off, but I felt secretly ecstatic. I really don't know why I was such a wimp.

---

these accounts were initiated and produced by patients without third-party influence. This literature can therefore be considered to be a genuine reflection of the patient's perspective on professional exploitation. This is in contrast to research performed using questionnaires and interviews, which impose a structure or pre-selected categories on the data.

Sadly, the profession has mostly either ignored these accounts or else treated them with hostility. For example, Ernesto Spinelli (2001, p. 161), a former Professor of Psychotherapy at Regent's College, London, described this genre as: 'a developing category of psychotherapeutically focused texts written by ex-clients: the "read how psychotherapy messed me up, how awful (or evil) it is" genre'. The profession's reaction to Rosie Alexander's (1995) book about her experience of non-sexual exploitation in psychotherapy was particularly hostile, as exemplified by the title of a review in *Counseling News* (Davis, 1996) – 'Rosie in Horrorland'. In her own reflections on publishing this work, Alexander described how her intention of initiating a debate on the subject came to nothing. She stated: 'any client daring to question what was being done to them in the name of therapy risks having their criticisms dismissed as ignorant lay presumption or even as a further indication of their psychological disorder' (Alexander, 2003, p. 291).

Using patient literature to understand sexualised therapies

My own research looked at 30 published self-authored accounts of unsatisfactory psychotherapy treatments. In 15, the patients experienced some significant sexualisation of the therapy. All of these cases involved a female patient and a male therapist. Accounts were examined using the qualitative, inductive methods of categorisation analysis (Lepper, 2000) and grounded theory (Strauss & Corbin, 1998). This approach enabled the study to focus on the patient's perception of those actions that both preceded and constituted the experience of exploitation.

Factors associated with the development of a sexualised relationship proved remarkably consistent. Of all the factors identified, therapist self-disclosure emerged as the most frequent and significant action preceding a sexually exploitative therapy. This was followed by other boundary breaches, the most common of which were:

- extending the sessions
- offering hugs or hand holding
- meeting in social contexts
- offering telephone contact between sessions
- giving gifts.

None of these actions was, however, implicated as consistently as disclosures. Understanding more about the impact of therapist disclosures on the patient was considered particularly important because of its relevance to ordinary practice.

Because the majority of practitioners would recognise that to reveal explicit sexual fantasies or sexual experiences would not be in the patient's interest, the more 'ordinary' type of disclosures that emerged are discussed here in more detail. It should also be made clear that patients did not suggest that all disclosures were unhelpful; in fact, many stated that brief disclosures that normalised the patient's situation could be useful. Problematic disclosures were categorised as *seductive* disclosures, the most commonly occurring of which were:

- self-enhancing disclosures – those that focused on the therapist's professional standing, achievements, superior personality traits, popularity and so on
- disclosures about feelings for the patient, particularly those focusing on the patient's attractiveness
- disclosures emphasising commonalities, leading to 'soul mate'-type implications, often conveyed with an observation about the pair's unique capacity for mutual understanding
- disclosures about how the therapist would treat the patient if he were her partner
- revelations about unsatisfactory aspects of the therapist's personal life, especially those relating to marital problems
- disclosures providing evidence that the therapist was treating the patient differently from other patients
- disclosures that the patient felt obliged to keep secret in order to protect the therapist.

Patients emphasised that these disclosures were frequently made in a very subtle way and retrospective reflections suggested that this added to the feeling of confusion and disempowerment that they generated. For example, a self-enhancing disclosure might be given when apologising for an absence, the therapist telling the patient that he had been pressed to speak at an international conference and it would cause great disappointment if he did not accept.

One client, 'Dr K', described the negative impact that accrued from her therapist using her sexual fantasies as 'springboards for editorializing about how a man *should* treat me, how *he* would treat me if he could' (quoted by Gabbard & Lester, 1995, p. 139; see also Box 2.2). Disclosures about the patient's attractiveness would also often initially be given indirectly. For example, Adams (2008, p. 124) recounts how she 'noted that a bus driver had let me on the bus without payment. To this he put his hand to his mouth and whispered "I bet he fancied you"'. The feeling of disempowerment was summed up well by one patient who commented 'I felt confused about how to process this information but also guilty about having noticed it'.

Gabbard & Lester (1995, p. 51) give a good explanation of why *any* indication on the part of the therapist of sexual feelings about the patient can be experienced in a profoundly negative way:

Disclosure of erotic countertransference usually has a different meaning for the patient from other feelings in the analyst. It may overwhelm and confuse the patient. It may threaten the patient with the inherent link between sexual feelings and action. And it frequently leads to a collapse of the analytic space because the concrete has replaced the symbolic.

Effects on the patient

Professionals often find it difficult to understand how disclosures of the type discussed above can have such a profoundly negative impact on the

---

Box 2.2 'It made me feel special'

The following extract is from the case of 'Dr K' (Gabbard & Lester, 1995).

When he shared his personal thoughts and reflections with me, they felt like secret gifts. I had understood that an analyst was like a blank screen. He was somewhat neutral but was not blank. He sometimes told me vignettes from his life. I felt special, as if I knew things about him that others did not. I felt he was giving me presents. They felt a bit like contraband. I would jealously and a bit guiltily guard those presents of self-revelation. I would never talk about him to anyone outside analysis, never reveal the things he told me. That made them all the more precious; furthermore, it made me feel special and secretly loyal to him. He and I had a little secret life. None of this was voiced by me, nor raised by him for inspection.

patient. The following elements, found in almost every account, help to explain why.

- *Elation*. The patient experiences an overwhelming feeling of 'specialness' as a result of the disclosures.
- *Transcendence*. The feeling of 'specialness' has a transcendent effect that appears to make the problems that brought the patient into therapy disappear.
- *Idealisation*. Because the transcendence is so closely related to the person of the therapist, the patient becomes bonded to the therapist and is then compelled to maintain the relationship at all costs.
- *Dependency*. The therapist quite literally becomes more important to the patient than anything else in her life.

More about the particular impact of this sequence of events was understood by paying close attention to the language used by patients. It was remarkably consistent and centred on a variety of adjectives associated with denying ordinary life. These images were predominantly magical, spiritual or pharmaceutical. Because the problems that had brought the patient into therapy seemed to disappear, it was very compelling and explained the patient's desire to suppress any anxieties about the professional's actions or motive. Several examples are given in order to emphasise the consistency of the imagery used:

I was swept up in something quite out of my control. I adored and worshipped him; he was the most wonderful person I had ever met. (Matteson, 2008, p. 54)

[The feeling was] so powerful as to become quasi-hallucinogenic. (Hellewell, 2006, p. 69)

By then the air felt so sweet and sexy I felt kissed by angels.... I was staggered by the magnificent light our mutual inflation seemed to shed on the psyche. (Anonymous, 2005, p. 671)

I lived and would have died for him; his love had saved me and I worshipped him; to be in his light was healing; no pain would have been too much to bear for him. (Nash, 2002, p. 4)

These quotations show how extreme and mystical the experience could become. The language evoked a feeling of the sublime and the religious imagery alluded to the notion of the therapist as 'saviour'. Dr K (Gabbard & Lester, 1995, p. 132) described the specific connection with the personality of the therapist particularly well in her account of her own experience of a seductive therapy. In describing how her psychological needs felt met, she stated 'a thirst never quenched was now being slaked. And perhaps most important, I felt it was being slaked by *him*. Not by the process. Not by something in me.' The therapist therefore became the catalyst and as such became utterly indispensable. In addition, there was the knowledge (conscious or unconscious) that puncturing the idealisation could precipitate a return to problems that had been so effectively deleted.

In every case, however, this phenomenon was ultimately profoundly debilitating and psychologically devastating.

Transference implications

In thinking about this phenomenon in theoretical terms, the idealisation described above was clearly 'transference' (in psychoanalytic terms, how feelings or longings about people from the past are transferred onto people in the present). Although patients did not usually use the word 'transference', the concept was implicitly evoked in descriptions that alluded to the lack of ordinary correspondence between the emotional experience and rational feelings about the person. A particularly common example was the confusion of being attracted to the professional, even though there was also a feeling of repulsion. For example, Adams (2008, p. 125) stated: 'I could not stop obsessively thinking about him and could not understand my feelings. He was 18 years older than me, had greasy hair, smelt unpleasantly of body odour and had a long unkempt beard.'

The idealising transference clearly puts the therapist in a very powerful position and it is not difficult to see how some professionals may be tempted to encourage the phenomenon, especially if operating from a narcissistic position. The therapist may even believe that the relationship *is* 'special' and that the feelings are real. Furthermore, he may convince himself that it is in the patient's interest, as evidenced by the improvement in her condition. In this way both patient and therapist conspire in its flourishing: the patient feels she has transcended her troubles; the therapist finds it difficult to give up the gratification.

Once this kind of idealisation and dependency are established, the relationship can very easily move from sexualised to sexual. Gabbard & Lester (1995) and Schoener *et al* (1989) describe the various kinds of sexual relations that are likely to develop. These range from situations that mimic an ordinary mutual relationship to those which take place only during the therapy hour and often consist of masturbatory acts performed on the therapist.

Wider impact on the patient

Retrospective accounts by patients suggested that the infantile state of mind that had arisen as a result of the regression and dependency was often taken out of the consulting room, to the detriment of other relationships. The consequence, in many cases, was that the therapeutic relationship became pre-eminent and interest in anything other than therapy vanished. Alexander (2003, p. 294) referred to this kind of dependency as 'enslavement'. Many patients described how the therapist encouraged them to regard therapy as the most important thing in their life and, as other relationships deteriorated, it actually became so.

In most cases the idealisation continued until the therapist broke the relationship, whether through boredom or fright at the disintegrating effect it was having on the patient's life outside the therapy. This not only left the patient feeling abandoned and betrayed but precipitated a return of the problems that had taken her into therapy in the first place. At this point the reality of the exploitation typically overwhelmed the patient. Almost all reported feeling unbearable distress. Many became suicidal. In almost all cases the feelings were complex and confusing, not least because most patients felt some degree of responsibility.

Therapists reacted almost invariably by pathologising the patient and it was not uncommon for them to alter their patient notes or to make retrospective notes detailing seductive behaviour on the part of the patient. In the majority of cases the patient was also ascribed borderline personality traits and therapists would often note the effect the patient had on their own mental health. Patients also reported collusion between colleagues. Several commented on how general practitioners and other professionals suddenly insisted on a chaperone being present.

In terms of symptoms, the literature details what Pope (1989) refers to as 'therapist–patient sex syndrome'. The symptoms reported by Pope and others corroborate those that emerged from patients' accounts. They included: return or worsening of original symptoms, uncontrollable mood swings, self-harming behaviour, depleted self-esteem, difficulties in concentrating, anxiety, depression, flashbacks to the therapy, reclusive behaviour and hypervigilance.

Prevention

I suggest that prevention falls into three main categories: patient information, professional practice and institutional responsibility.

Patient engagement

More information should be given to patients about unacceptable practices. The strangeness and unfamiliarity of the 'rules' governing the process of psychotherapy serve to disempower the patient. A particular difficulty is that the patient is unable to compare therapy to any other relationship, which makes aberrant practices difficult both to identify and to contest. As a result, common-sense intuition is often subordinated to the professional's assumed knowledge. The inherent asymmetrical nature of the relationship can also make the patient reluctant to confront or question the professional. Patients describe their sense of frustration at not having enough information or recourse to consultation to 'check out' what is happening. They link this directly with their own failure to act and to feelings of disempowerment as the treatment progresses. A list of unacceptable practices, including the more subtle aspects of disclosure, should therefore be given to patients at the start of therapy. It is also helpful for a patient to be given the contact details of another professional with whom they can discuss any concerns, on an informal basis, *as they arise*. If concerns were dealt with promptly, before the situation becomes acrimonious, much damage and many complaints could be prevented.

Informed consent is a concept that most therapists do not regard as relevant to psychotherapy. Patients who developed an idealising transference were, however, very clear that they should have been warned that this was a possibility before the therapy began. Several patients in the study compared the incapacitating effects of the transference to the side-effects of a drug. They observed that if they had been given a drug which could incapacitate them to the same extent the clinician would have had a duty to inform them.

Professional practice

Philosophers from Aristotle to Kant have emphasised that ethical competence is *not* intrinsic but is a skill that needs to be cultivated and practised. This means striving for transparency and constantly questioning both individual practices and the practices of institutions. The philosopher Zygmunt Bauman (1993, p. 80) suggests that anxiety is necessary in ethical practice and sums this up well in suggesting that: 'The moral self is always haunted by the suspicion that it is not moral enough'.

This 'anxiety' must focus on those aspects of practice that may encourage regression, dependency and idealisation. In particular, practitioners must be aware of how some profoundly unhelpful interactions can masquerade as a 'cure'. The psychoanalyst Jonathan Lear (2003, p. 100) is unusual in raising this. He states that if we 'use the positive transference rather than analyse it, we can achieve results that, on the surface at least, look rather decisive. Our patients will tell us they feel increased emotional freedom and marvel at our abilities as analysts.'

In order to ensure that this does not happen, clinicians need to discuss any subtle indications of idealisation *as they arise*. The professional needs to be aware that if such idealisation is not interpreted, these feelings can become fixed and intractable. An important opportunity for thinking about the 'real' meaning of the transference will also be lost. Sandner (1995, p. 4) – quoted by Anonymous (2005, p. 666) – very succinctly summarises this as 'ego inflation', which can lead to a temptation to 'neglect the transference'.

Institutional responsibility

Institutions need to take a 'zero tolerance' attitude to the sexualisation of therapy. Many institutions still turn a blind eye to the fact that particular practitioners exploit patients and they strive to ensure that the outcome of professional conduct hearings is kept secret. A surprising and consistent finding is that exploitative practitioners are often charismatic individuals who have status and standing within the institution to which they belong (Gabbard & Lester, 1995, p. 132). Schoener *et al* take a very non-compromising view regarding both institutions and individuals who are 'bystanders' of abuse in declaring: 'There is no "middle ground". One is either part of the problem or part of the solution. To fail to take action is the ultimate crime of silence' (Schoener *et al*, 1989, p. 4).

There is, however, a lack of transparency in psychotherapy organisations, as evidenced by a survey I undertook on the accessibility of codes of ethics. The websites of 70 institutional members of the United Kingdom Council for Psychotherapy (UKCP) were surveyed and 36% were found to make no reference to the existence of a code of ethics or complaints process; 74% did not make their code available on their website; 97% did not acknowledge that therapy could be problematic. Of the 74% that did not make their code available on their website, a further 17% of them did not send their code when it was requested. A code of ethics is often the only information the patient has access to about ethical standards. These figures therefore indicate the extent to which complacency and opacity resides at the heart of institutional attitudes to ethical practice in psychotherapy.

Treatment needs following exploitation

As might be expected, patients who present after experiencing professional abuse can have extremely complex further treatment needs. Schoener and his colleagues at the Walk-In Counseling Center (WICC) in Minneapolis have specialised in treating professional abuse since 1974, when they began to devote specific resources to the problem. Their seminal work, *Psycho-therapists' Sexual Involvement with Clients: Intervention and Prevention* (Schoener *et al*, 1989) clearly sets out the parameters of the problem and gives detailed advice on all aspects of treatment. In tackling this question of treatment, I draw on the experience of Schoener and his colleagues as well of my own experience of treating patients who have suffered professional abuse.

The treating therapist must consider not only how the patient has been adversely affected by this experience but also that the problems which took the patient into therapy will not have been addressed. As discussed above, one of the compelling aspects of the sexualised relationship is that problems seem to disappear magically and so are never addressed, even though the therapy may have cost thousands of pounds and lasted for many years. Patients often focus on this aspect of the exploitation and find the lost opportunity particularly difficult to come to terms with, sometimes even more so than the sexual abuse.

Transference considerations are likely to be paramount for the treating therapist because the patient may experience ordinary actions as seductive. For example, agreeing to reschedule a session at the patient's request may serve as a reminder of previous 'special treatment'. The consulting room may also become the repository of projections and feelings transferred from the previous therapy. For instance, everyday objects may be treated with suspicion or take on a sinister meaning (Devereux, 2006). I have found it helpful to address these issues as they arise in a sensitive, conversational manner which respects the patient's perspective but gently teases out the transference. Some patients are very aware of the transference and are adept at interpreting it for themselves as it arises.

Therapists also need to be able to let patients develop a sense of trust in the process and to accept the fact that these patients will come to therapy with a depleted capacity to trust professionals. This is an entirely appropriate adaptive response. Despite this, many patients report experiencing adverse reactions from therapists who inappropriately 'demand' trust as a precondition to 'the therapy working'.

Patients report two dominant types of countertransference reactions in treating therapists. First, some therapists are extremely defensive, as if they are on constant alert for any indication that the patient will complain about them. Patients have also reported experiencing very rigid boundaries, which feel punitive and discriminatory rather than containing. A common example is for therapists in private practice to suggest that the patient needs the containment of an institutional setting, which leaves the patient feeling stigmatised.

Second, the converse countertransference response is for therapists to feel compelled to prove to the patient that they are not abusive. In their desire to give the patient a restorative experience they may abandon their usual analytic neutrality and treat the patient in a special way. A common example is to refer to the abusive therapist in a pejorative manner in an effort to convince the patient that they are 'on their side'. Schoener *et al* (1989) suggest that while it may be important for the treating therapist to begin by making it clear that the previous treatment was abusive, it is not helpful to continue to make such references. This is because these patients need the space to process their own feelings, without having to take into account the therapist's.

Patients are often extremely angry about the previous exploitation but their feelings about the abusive professional can also be very confused. Both shame and guilt are very common. Shame is most often associated with the fact that patients may feel they have 'allowed' this to happen. Profound feelings of guilt are associated with many factors, ranging from the effect the abuse has had on those close to them, to feeling that they have betrayed the therapist. Feelings of paranoia can also occur, particularly with respect to feeling that the therapist will know the patient has disclosed the abuse. I have treated patients who were convinced that the therapist had bugged my consulting room and would know that they were disclosing the abuse.

The propensity to self-harm once the abuse is over is not uncommon, even when there was no history of this. The self-harm is not always obvious and may take the form of a repetition of some traumatic aspect of the therapy. For example, patients report becoming promiscuous for the first time in their life or financially irresponsible.

Most patients are in great need of a facilitating space in which to process the trauma, but hypervigilance and intrusive transferences can make this difficult to achieve. In such cases I have found eye movement desensitisation reprogramming (EMDR) to be a particularly effective treatment; the National Institute of Health and Clinical Excellence (2005) recommends this for the treatment of post-traumatic stress disorder (PTSD). Because this intervention is predictable and process driven it can be particularly effective with those patients in whom a depleted capacity to trust makes it difficult to get the therapy started.

The effect of a complaints process on the therapy

As part of seeking therapy, patients often want to explore the various forms of redress available to them. Options include mediation, making a complaint to the therapist's professional organisation, making a complaint to the health authority or civil action for negligence. Again, treating therapists can react to this in polarised ways. Some take on the authority of moral experts and coerce patients into taking action. This is often based on a very naive view of what a complaints process involves. A complaints process may take years to complete, during which time the patient may feel that her life has been put on hold. The decision about whether to make a complaint must be based purely on the best interests of the patient. Patients must be supported in their decision, without being burdened with the notion that they have a responsibility to society.

If the patient does decide to make a complaint it is important for the treating therapist to bear in mind the way this is likely to affect treatment. Some complaints' processes are conducted so badly that they can be experienced as a recapitulation of the worst aspects of the therapy. As Gabbard & Lester (1995, p. 181) stated, if patients 'have the courage to step forward and report details of their analyst's boundary violations, they are often treated with reactions ranging from contempt to minimization to defensive aloofness'. This is especially so if the therapist is a psychotherapist rather than a psychiatrist or psychologist. This is because psychotherapists have resisted state regulation. Complaints to the largest voluntary regulator, UKCP, often take years to complete and patients are required to represent themselves (or pay for legal representation) against a therapist whose insurance company is likely to provide a barrister. Furthermore, criminal standards of proof are commonly used and panels may comprise only the therapist's close colleagues. One UKCP organisation (The Guild of Psychotherapists) even claims the right to make the patient responsible for the ethics panel's costs if the complaint is not upheld, adding greatly to the stress of a complaints process.

In practical terms, the treating therapist will also need to consider the fact that the patient's notes may need to be disclosed in the case of criminal or civil action. It is essential for the therapist to think about how this might affect the patient's freedom of expression: many patients fear that comments in notes may be distorted and so withhold important information from the treating therapist. As a way of alleviating this, the therapist might consider offering copies of the notes after each session.

Some therapists do not want to get involved in giving witness statements. They believe that by refusing they are behaving in a neutral manner and claim to do so in the interests of preserving the therapy. When a therapist (or any other person) refuses to give a witness statement, however, he or she is merely colluding with the abuse. It is difficult to overemphasise how profoundly distressing and undermining this can be for the patient. Elie Wiesel, the Nobel Peace Prize laureate, referred to this as 'bystanding'. He declared that 'what hurts the victim most is not the cruelty of the oppressor, but the silence of the bystander' (quoted in Rittner & Meyers, 1986, p. 2).

Conclusion

This chapter has shown how profound and devastating the consequences of sexual abuse by healthcare professionals can be. By putting the emphasis on factors that precede sexual abuse, the aim has been to alert practitioners to the dangers of self-enhancing disclosures and the temptation to encourage idealisation, regression and dependency. A particular objective has been to highlight the complacency that can exist within institutions in relation to abusive practices. This is exemplified by lengthy complaints processes that fail to deliver proper sanctions, as well as a general attitude of indifference to the needs of the complainant. Patients who have been subjected to professional abuse need to be supported and treated in a manner that takes into account the additional difficulties that accrue from having to re-engage with a professional. The treating therapist must therefore consider how he or she can best provide a facilitating space so that the patient has a restorative experience of psychotherapy and can begin to re-establish an appropriate sense of trust.

References

Adams, J. (2008) *Broken Boundaries: Sexual and Non-sexual Boundary Violations in the Psychological Therapies*. Witness.

Alexander, R. (1995) *Folie a Deux*. Free Association Press.

Alexander, R. (2003) A client's wish for the future. In *Ethically Challenged Professions: Enabling Innovation and Diversity in Psychotherapy and Counselling* (eds Y. Bates & R. House), pp. 291–297. PCCS Books.

Anonymous (2005) The unfolding and healing of analytic boundary violations: personal, clinical and cultural considerations. *Journal of Analytical Psychology*, **50**, 661–691.

Bates, C. & Brodsky, A. (1988) *Sex in the Therapy Hour*. Guilford Press.

Bauman, Z. (1993) *Postmodern Ethics*. Blackwell.

Casemore, R. (2001) *Surviving Complaints Against Counsellors and Psychotherapists*. PCCS Books.

Davis, L. (1996) 'Rosie in Horrorland': review of Alexander's *Folie a Deux*. *Counseling News*, March, p. 30.

Devereux, D. (2006) Enactment: some thoughts about the therapist's contribution. *British Journal of Psychotherapy*, **22**, 497–508.

Freeman, L. & Roy, J. (1976) *Betrayal*. Stein and Day.

Gabbard, G. O. & Lester, E. (1995) *Boundaries and Boundary Violations in Psychoanalysis*. American Psychiatric Publishing.

Guild of Psychotherapists (2005) *Code of Ethics*. Online at www.guildofpsychotherapists.org.uk (accessed 12 November 2009).

Hellewell, M. (2006) The client says not. In *Shouldn't I Be Feeling Better By Now? Client Views of Therapy* (ed. Y. Bates). Palgrave Macmillan.

Lear, J. (2003) *Therapeutic Action: An Earnest Plea for Irony*. Other Press.

Lepper, G. (2000) *Categories in Text and Talk*. Sage.

Matteson, M. (2008) *Broken Boundaries: Sexual and Non-Sexual Boundary Violations in the Psychological Therapies*. Witness.

Nash, P. (2002) *Survivors Forum Newsletter, 13*. Survivors Forum.

National Institute of Health and Clinical Excellence (2005) *Post-Traumatic Stress Disorder (PTSD)* (CG26). Online at http://guidance.nice.org.uk (accessed 12 November 2009).

Plasil, E. (1985) *Therapist*. St Martin's Press.

Pope, K. S. (1989) Therapist–patient sex syndrome: a guide for attorneys and subsequent therapists to assessing damage. In *Sexual Exploitation in Professional Relationships* (ed. G. Gabbard), pp. 39–55. American Psychiatric Press.

Rittner, C. & Meyers, S. (1986) *Courage to Care – Rescuers of Jews During the Holocaust*. New York University Press.

Sandner, D. (1995) Bipolar split in analytical psychology. Address at the IXth Congress for Analytical Psychology, Zurich, Switzerland.

Schoener, G., Milgrom, J., Gonsiorek, J., *et al* (1989) *Psychotherapists' Sexual Involvement with Clients: Intervention and Prevention*. Minneapolis, MN: Walk-In Counseling Center.

Spinelli, E. (2001) *The Mirror and the Hammer*. Continuum.

Strauss, A. & Corbin, J. (1998) *Basics of Qualitative Research*. Sage.

CHAPTER 3

Teaching ethics and ethical behaviour to medical students

Peter Haughton, Claire Spake and Ngozi Chukwudi

Overview

Patients want and need competent doctors. Competency comes through learning, practice and experience. It is validated by others who already possess the requisite skills and knowledge. It is this validation that is a key component of becoming and being a professional. Although there is an assumption that it can, the question is whether or not appropriate behaviour can be taught to those training to be doctors. We report here the various measures currently used for such teaching, and draw on the evidence and our combined experience as a teacher of medical ethics and law, and as clinical medical students. This chapter looks at what is currently being taught and its effectiveness in relation to clinical ethical competency.

Background to the teaching of medical ethics in UK medical schools

It has only been in the past 20 years or so that ethics as a subject in its own right has been formally taught in UK medical schools. Although there had earlier been enthusiasts making the case for the inclusion of formal teaching of ethics and law within the curriculum (see below), a key catalyst for change in the UK was the publication in 1987 of the Pond report (Boyd, 1987), followed in 1993 by *Tomorrow's Doctors*, published by the General Medical Council (GMC, 1993), which set out in broad terms what was expected of medical schools in the training of medical students. The teaching of medical ethics and the acquiring of appropriate behaviour were specifically mentioned. Since medical schools had to demonstrate that they met the terms of the GMC's requirements, room was made in a crowded syllabus for some ethics teaching. The content of what might be taught emerged through a consensus statement (see Box 3.1). This was

---

Box 3.1 Teaching and assessing ethics and law within medical education: a model for the core curriculum

The following 12 topics were identified as core to the teaching and assessment of ethics and law within the medical curriculum in a consensus statement by teachers of medical ethics and law in UK medical schools (Anonymous, 1998):

- Informed consent and refusal of treatment
- The clinical relationship – truthfulness, trust and good communication
- Confidentiality and good clinical practice
- Medical research
- Human reproduction
- The 'new genetics'
- Children
- Mental disorders and disabilities
- Life, death, dying and killing
- Vulnerabilities created by the duties of doctors and medical students
- Resource allocation
- Rights.

---

revisited under the auspices of the Institute of Medical Ethics (Stirrat *et al*, 2010). The latest editions of the GMC's *Tomorrow's Doctors* (2009*a*) and *Medical Students: Professional Values and Fitness to Practise* (2009*b*) will bring about further change to the medical schools' curriculum.

The introduction of medical ethics as a core component of the undergraduate curriculum has not been without opposition. Hope (1998) addressed the three principal reasons behind the resistance. Medical ethics education was deemed:

1   trivial – the resolution of ethical dilemmas is generally obvious
2   redundant – teaching of ethics is not necessary, as this is done in a clinical context
3   impossible – as it is argued that one cannot be taught moral attitudes and character.

Advocates of a medical ethics programme contested these arguments on the grounds of the overriding effectiveness of ethics teaching for good medical practice, although this claim was difficult to substantiate. Early inroads in America are described by McElhinney & Pellegrino (1982). What duly followed was the gradual development of medical ethics within the medical education system (Jacobson *et al*, 1989) and the assertion, by practising clinicians, of clinical medical ethics as a vital clinical skill (Kern *et al*, 1985). In addition, students exposed to ethics training in their preclinical years desired its continuation into their clinical training (Howe, 1987). Miles *et al* (1989) provided an authoritative review regarding medical

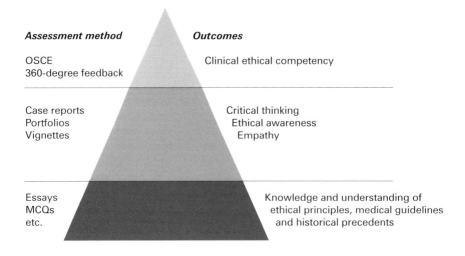

Fig. 3.1 The ascending pyramid illustrating the aims of medical ethics education (Campbell *et al*, 2007). OSCE, objective structured clinical examination; MCQs, multiple-choice questions.

ethics education in the USA, and therein proposed five desirable premises of medical ethics education:

ethics education should (1) be conceptually coherent, (2) be vertically and horizontally integrated through preclinical and clinical training, (3) be multidisciplinary, (4) be academically rigorous, and (5) demonstrate humane and value-conscious medical practice.

These premises were designed to assist the teaching, structure and programme of medical ethics, but implementation was problematic.

A conference held by the Institute of Medical Ethics, the British Medical Association and the Higher Education Academy Subject Centre for Medicine, Dentistry and Veterinary Medicine in 2006 revisited the core consensus of 1998 and formulated a fresh set of the proposed aims of medical ethics education. Knowledge, habituation and action were identified as three distinct levels (the primary aims of medical ethics education), illustrated as an ascending pyramid in Fig. 3.1. How these aims interlink can be summed up by the quote 'knowledge is needed for habituation [*sic*], to shape the mould within which a student behaves so that there emerges action of a kind that is clinically appropriate and effective' (Campbell *et al*, 2007). Knowledge, as well as understanding, consists of specifically ethical principles, medical guidelines and historical precedents. This is the initial learning objective of medical ethics education and the suggested assessment method of this would be essays, multiple-choice questions (MCQs) or various adaptations to assess the understanding of the ethical theoretical concepts. 'Habituation' – defined here as accustoming students to think critically, demonstrate ethical awareness in the clinical context and empathise with patients by frequent repetition or prolonged exposure – is the next level in this hierarchy. At this stage students are assessed by case reports, as these provide opportunity for students to reflect on ethical dilemmas in clinical settings and analyse the appropriate course of action. The writing of portfolios and case vignettes demonstrates students' development and their perception of the diverse ethical questions that arise in given situations. A potential flaw with the use of clinical vignettes is what is referred to as the 'quandary ethics' approach, where there is the tendency to neglect the ethical dimensions of everyday medical encounters and instead focus on dramatic, 'life and death' cases. At the top of this pyramid lies action, and the indicated desired outcome of medical ethics education is clinical ethical competency (Campbell *et al*, 2007).

The GMC's recommendations for medical ethics as part of the core medical curriculum monitored by its regular visits to medical schools have shifted the historical dilemma from *whether* to include medical ethics into the curriculum to *how* best to do this with regard to teaching style and content (Hope, 1998). As a teacher of medical ethics, it is relatively easy to demonstrate the first step of the pyramid model above. The knowledge and its application can be, and are, tested in the form of short-answer questions based around clinical situations that the student might have been expected to have encountered. A difficulty that arises is the artificiality of assessment. The answer that students give to the question 'What would you do and why?' under examination conditions may be very different from what they might do in reality. A parallel might be drawn between those undergoing their driving test and their subsequent driving. Likewise, medical students in objective structured clinical examinations (OSCEs) will interact with patients, both real and simulated, in a manner that they think is appropriate for the examination, to show that they have taken on the skills learnt from the classroom, but not necessarily what they have acquired from the ward round.

Teaching medical ethics

The 1998 consensus statement left the autonomy of how to teach these topics to the individual medical schools. Lectures and small-group sessions are most commonly used individually or in conjunction. Using the context of real cases in which students are involved is ideal (Loewy, 1986). Small-group teaching enables adequate discussion of cases, which would prove difficult in large classes. A study by Self *et al* (1998) showed that small-group discussion significantly increases moral reasoning skills – a fundamental component of moral development. This prompts subsequent consideration of the identifiable effects of ethics education.

Much of the initial teaching was the application of ethical principles to clinical case studies. This principle approach stemmed from the hugely influential work of Beauchamp & Childress (1978), popularised in the UK largely by Professor Raanan Gillon, through his editorship of the *Journal of Medical Ethics* and other writing (Gillon, 1985; Gillon & Lloyd 1994).

The superficial beauty of the principle approach was its simplicity. Complex clinical problems could have the ethical/moral component analysed through the consideration of four principles (respect for autonomy, non-maleficence, beneficence and justice) and the right course of action could be determined. Medical students could learn the four principles and apply them to the various clinical problems set before them. It was as if the principles could be put into the doctor's medical bag and drawn upon whenever a moral problem was encountered. Additional topics, such as obtaining consent, assessing competence, keeping confidentiality and the nature of the doctor–patient relationship would be taught and explored. The weakness was the misapprehension that all doctors needed to do was to learn and apply these four principles. In other words, there was a danger of 'dumbing down' and reducing medical ethics to this 'principlist' approach and believing that the subject had been taught.

The programme run at King's College London (by the first author) is based on Campbell's model above. In the first 2 years all medical students attend lectures, which are followed by 'break-out' groups. The aim of these sessions is to inculcate the various concepts critical to good clinical practice. The students are encouraged to take them on board through the use of small facilitated discussion groups using clinical case studies. The overall aim of this programme is to prepare the students for the greater clinical component of their studies. There is also a change from directed learning (preclinical) to self-directed learning (clinical). In the clinical years there are opportunities for students to take time out of their studies in order to reflect on the ethical issues that they have encountered.

A similar pattern is used on the full-time year-long intercalated BSc in medical ethics and law at King's College. The first semester is predominantly taught through extensive guided reading and interactive seminars. During the second semester the students attend a wide variety of clinical placements. Compulsory dedicated time is given each week for the students to reflect on their experiences. They are encouraged to make links between ethical theory and practice, and to discover common problems in different areas of medical practice. The links between theory and practice are explored. Within the confines of a closed, facilitated discussion group the students gain confidence in formulating the components of good clinical practice. Initially the students struggle with these groups, partly because they are not used to this type of learning and partly because they have not experienced the intimacy of such focused attention. Yet, from student feedback, it is these facilitated reflective sessions that are the most memorable and valued. It is unfortunate that such quality time for clinical reflection is not made available within the core curriculum.

The effects of medical ethics education

There is some evidence that exposure to medical ethics teaching leads to greater ethical sensitivity in the clinical context. For example, a preliminary study by Hebert *et al* (1992) at the University of Toronto demonstrated an increase in ethical sensitivity between the first and second year of medical school, by measuring students' ability to identify ethical issues in four clinical vignettes. Goldie *et al* (2001) also showed, by looking at the outcomes of the Glasgow University Medical School curriculum, that a first-year group exposed to ethics training, in comparison with a control group who had not been exposed, had an enhanced capacity to make ethical judgements consistent with experts. This tool of assessment was called the 'consensus professional judgement'. A significant benefit of medical ethics teaching is demonstrated as an improvement in moral reasoning (Self *et al*, 1989) and the format of this teaching that most significantly contributes to this is small-group ethics teaching (Goldie *et al*, 2002). Students exposed to 20 hours or more of small-group case-study ethics teaching demonstrated a significant increase in scores for moral reasoning (Self *et al*, 1998). In addition, there is also a positive impact, shown in the students in year 1 with whom this was the primary format in a cohort study for the University of Glasgow Medical School (Goldie *et al*, 2004). The results of small-group ethical teaching may be attributed to the fact that this forum provides students with an opportunity to explore and express their concerns (Osborne & Martin, 1989). A pertinent study by Johnston & Haughton (2007) considering the perception of medical students regarding their ethics teaching highlighted a student penchant for small-group teaching, also known as break-out sessions, as they enable vital ethical discussion, debate and ownership of the taught material.

Unfortunately, there is evidence which suggests that the experience of clinical teaching nullifies the initial ethical sensitivity that has been inculcated in the early part of a medical student's education. In the same study cited above by Hebert *et al* (1992) a decrease in ethical sensitivity was found in the years following undergraduate medical training, which was assumed to result from a lack of reinforcement in the clinical years. This loss in ethical sensitivity in the clinical ('cynical') years is corroborated by other studies (Akabayashi *et al*, 2004; Goldie *et al*, 2004). A clinical culture that undermines and devalues ethics subsequently results in a reversal of the intended outcomes of first-year medical ethics education.

Self *et al* (1989) actually noted a regression in the scores for moral reasoning among students taught by lectures, with a simultaneous rise in scores among small-group cohorts, possibly due to a lack of cognitive dissonance and engagement promoted by the lecture format. In similar fashion, Cowley (2008) warns against utilising medical ethics as one would a scientific body of knowledge as 'there is a real risk that spurious technocratic jargon will be deployed by teacher and student alike in the futile search for intellectual respectability'. However, there is a tendency for students to want definite answers, even in ethics (Hope, 1998). The 'hidden curriculum' may inhibit the development of moral reasoning, as suggested by Patenaude *et al* (2003); in their cohort study, Canadian medical students had demonstrated a decline in moral development at the end of their third year. The impact of the 'hidden curriculum' and whether ethics teaching is capable of overcoming it is reviewed below when considering the impact of medical ethics education in the production of morally acting health professionals.

Evaluating the impact of medical ethics education

From the published papers, it is evident that medical ethics education does have an impact, yet the tools used to measure and evaluate these effects are less than satisfactory. Savulescu *et al* (1999) argue for the need for a 'relevant, reliable and valid instrument to evaluate core critical thinking skills in medical ethics'. The establishment of such an instrument would provide greater evidence for the once ambiguous role of ethics as a key player in the core undergraduate curriculum. The critical question of whether ethics teaching has a measurable effect on the clinical activity of students exposed to it persists and Mitchell *et al* (1993) highlight the progression from the assessment of students' ethical knowledge base to the actual application of this knowledge, known as 'clinical ethical competence'.

In essence, it is clear that evaluation of medical ethics teaching is vital. However, there still prevails a methodological limitation where the validity and reliability of some of the instruments of evaluation are not fully established (Wong & Cheung, 2003). No 'gold standard' for ethics assessment has yet been validated (Goldie, 2000).

Medical ethics education and 'moral' health professionals

Some studies have shown that medical ethics education increases moral reasoning and sensitivity in those exposed to it. The illogical deduction is that this training is also capable of creating sound moral character. This, however, is considered an unrealistic expectation by Culver *et al* (1985), who dismissed it by proposing that the goal of medical ethics education is the development of knowledge and skills in those of *pre-existing* sound moral character. Thus moral character is *not* an outcome of medical ethics education. If this is the case, then can it be established whether there is a link between moral reasoning or sensitivity (identifiable outcomes of medical ethics education) and moral *action* in clinical practice? Some might argue simplistically that moral action is a sequential follow-on from ethical knowledge acquisition and habituation – as shown in Fig. 3.1. The counter-argument is provided in a sample of cohort studies which suggest counteracting influences that impede or cause a regression in ethical conduct despite adequate undergraduate medical ethics training. Acting in accordance to ingrained ethical principles may be difficult, as highlighted by Rosenbaum *et al* (2004), who conducted a qualitative study which revealed there are several sources of ethical conduct that exist for medical house officers. The ideals of ethical principles may be 'unattainable' when deliberating between two competing professional values, say autonomy and non-maleficence. McDougall (2009) narrates what he describes as '4 a.m. logic', which appears to be the common scenario where junior doctors come against great difficulties in 'aligning their actions with the values they reflectively embrace' owing to the various levels of coercion within pressurised hospital environments. However, an especially disconcerting finding is highlighted by Satterwhite *et al* (2000) as an 'ethical paradox'. This is where exposure to unethical situations, for example derogatory statements concerning patients, induces an acceptance of unethical conduct but with coexistent denial by those partaking in this that their traditional code of ethics has altered. The authors of this study proposed that there is in fact a transformation of the doctors' code of ethics so that it matches their behaviour, providing consistency between judgement and action. In other words, the ethics is reshaped to practice rather than being instrumental as a critique of practice.

In essence, it appears that there is much discouraging evidence concerning unethical behaviour irrespective of previous medical ethical training. These studies highlight the limitation of medical ethics education if it is restricted to the undergraduate realm within the 'walls of the classroom'. The findings from these studies lead to the consideration of the effect of the 'hidden curriculum'. This 'hidden curriculum' is essentially the external messages regarding what is 'good' and 'bad' clinical practice, derived from outside the formal ethics curriculum. These messages, rather than reinforcing the intended aims of medical ethics education, may be in direct conflict with it, resulting in moral relativism and cynicism (Hafferty & Franks, 1994). Acknowledgement of this hidden curriculum by medical ethics educators, and subsequently transcending it, may assist in assuring the guaranteed translation of moral reasoning into moral action. Rose & Rukstalis (2008) suggested that clinical mentoring can contribute to the transmission of ethics. If this is successfully incorporated into medical ethics education, it may be a tool for negating the deleterious effects of the hidden curriculum. A survey of Swedish medical schools conducted by Lynoe *et al* (2008) corroborates the benefits of mentorship in the form of role models, by indicating that increased interest in medical ethics is related to encounters with good clinical role models, and the inverse is true for poor role models.

It is clear that the subject matter of medical ethics and law is being taught in medical schools through a variety of methods. What is less clear is whether the teaching of the subject is instrumental in shaping clinical ethical competency. The change from the classroom to the clinic, from directed learning to more experiential learning, is a critical transformation. A number of factors undermine the good practice ideals inculcated in the early part of the course. Current clinicians may themselves lack confidence to tackle and articulate the ethical problems that they encounter. Students may feel powerless to challenge doctors when the students see dubious practice. There is a perception that clinical practice is 'real', whereas the classroom is artificial. The gulf between theory and practice is too wide for students to bridge, with the consequence that they cease to try. The case studies presented in Box 3.2, which arose from small-group discussions, illustrate this gulf between theory and practice. They describe two of the many examples of students' concerns brought to the first author's attention in the past year.

The 'hidden curriculum', illustrated by such examples, severely undermines the preparatory work of teachers of ethics and law in the preclinical phase of the medical course. By the very nature of these types of incident, actual numbers are hard to substantiate, yet we suspect that each clinical student on graduation could state a case that raises ethical concern. The medical school tries to address these matters, briefing students at the beginning of the clinical phase, but there is a general reluctance for students to respond or report.

Box 3.2 Medical students' ethical concerns: two case studies

1. A senior house officer asked by a final-year student on placement at a district general hospital why he decided on a career in medicine, in the context of drinks after work, replied 'It gives me the opportunity to examine prepubescent girls'.
   Comment. The student did nothing at the time as she was not sure whether she was having her 'leg pulled' and being provoked into reacting. It was only in the environment of a small-group setting following an interactive seminar on whistle-blowing that she was prepared to share this anecdote with medical school staff. Even then she did not name the individual or the hospital.

2. A final-year medical student (female) in theatre witnessed the surgeon (male) having simulated sex with the unconscious male patient, supposedly to the amuse-ment of the other people present, but to the disgust and horror of the medical student.
   Comment. It could be said that the wrongness of this behaviour does not need to be spelt out. And yet such behaviour displays a complete disregard of the patient as a person, turning the patient into an object on which the surgeon could express his warped sense of humour. What is of concern is that the medical student (and maybe other witnesses) felt powerless to do anything about it at the time. This incident came to light only in the context of a small-group discussion.

Box 3.3 A medical student reflects on the intensive BSc ethics teaching

The medical ethics and law intercalated BSc really opened my eyes to ethical and legal situations in the daily clinical environment. The medical school ought to appreciate that medical students will come across death, families dealing with bereavement and loss, and terminally ill patients, which are all harsh realities of a career in medicine but are still not explored in any great depth. There are insecurities over whether what you are witnessing *is* actually wrong or is it being overshadowed by the clinical experience and respect for the more senior doctor? There is little focus in the core curriculum on the benefits of whistle-blowing and the MBBS programme offers little guidance or support on this.

Before my BSc, I witnessed an appallingly insensitive breaking of a cancer diagnosis. When doing what I felt was the right thing – reporting to my personal tutor – the matter was not followed up and I did nothing further, which I regret. The reflective sessions held for the BSc, in which quality time was given over to explore the various dynamics of healthcare professionals' interactions with their patients, drew directly on observed experience; these were where our most informative learning took place. Is it perhaps ignorant to think that ethics cannot be taught, to believe that one's ethical mind cannot be developed? And is it arrogant to believe that you have all the right answers already? Having completed a BSc in clinical ethics I still don't have all the right answers, but I feel better prepared to tackle medical dilemmas. I found it empowering, knowing that I have the class group in which to discuss clinical issues. The BSc helped me to grow in confidence and improve skills of discussion and debate, to both listen *and* put my point across. I feel I am more receptive to the moral dilemmas I may not have even noticed before.

Conclusion

It would seem that teaching ethical behaviour to medical students may raise *awareness* of ethical sensitivities (Box 3.3) and therefore may *predispose* students to ethical conduct but, ultimately, it can never guarantee it. Any teaching may be undermined or reinforced by the exposure of students to unethical practice, the 'hidden curriculum', good or bad role models and room for safe reflection.

References

Akabayashi, A., Slingsby, B. T., Kai, I., *et al* (2004) The development of a brief and objective method of evaluating moral sensitivity and reasoning in medical students. *BMC Medical Ethics*, **5**, 1–7.

Anonymous (1998) Teaching medical ethics and law within medical education. A model for the UK core curriculum. Consensus statement by teachers of medical ethics and law in UK medical schools. *Journal of Medical Ethics*, **24**, 188–192.

Beauchamp, T. L. & Childress, J. F. (1978) *Principles of Biomedical Ethics*. Oxford University Press.

Boyd, K. M. (ed.) (1987) *Report of a Working Party on the Teaching of Medical Ethics* (the Pond report). IME.

Campbell, A. V., Chin, J. & Voo, T. (2007) How can we know that ethics education produces ethical doctors? *Medical Teacher*, **29**, 431–436.

Cowley, C. (2008) *Medical Ethics, Ordinary Concepts and Ordinary Lives.* Palgrave Macmillan.

Culver, C. M., Clouser, K. D., Gert, B., *et al* (1985) Basic curricular goals in medical ethics. *New England Journal of Medicine*, **312**, 253–256.

General Medical Council (1993) *Tomorrow's Doctors.* GMC.

General Medical Council (2009a) *Tomorrow's Doctors.* GMC.

General Medical Council (2009b) *Medical Students: Professional Values and Fitness to Practise.* GMC

Gillon, R. (1985) *Philosophical Medical Ethics.* Wiley.

Gillon, R. & Lloyd, A. (eds) (1994) *Principles of Healthcare Ethics.* Wiley.

Goldie, J. (2000) Review of ethics curricula in undergraduate medical education. *Medical Education*, **34**, 108–119.

Goldie, J., Schwartz, L., McConnachie, A., *et al* (2001) Impact of a new course on students' potential behaviour on encountering ethical dilemmas. *Medical Education*, **35**, 295–302.

Goldie, J., Schwartz, L., McConnachie, A., *et al* (2002) The impact of three years' ethics teaching, in an integrated medical curriculum, on students' proposed behaviour on meeting ethical dilemmas. *Medical Education*, **36**, 489–497.

Goldie, J., Schwartz, L., McConnachie, A., *et al* (2004) The impact of a modern medical curriculum on students' proposed behaviour on meeting ethical dilemmas. *Medical Education*, **38**, 942–949.

Hafferty, F. W. & Franks, R. (1994) The hidden curriculum, ethics teaching and the structure of medical education. *Academic Medicine*, **69**, 861–871.

Hebert, P. C., Meslin, E. M. & Dunn, E. V. (1992) Measuring the ethical sensitivity of medical students: a study at the University of Toronto. *Journal of Medical Ethics*, **18**, 142–147.

Hope, T. (1998) Ethics and law for medical students: the core curriculum. *Journal of Medical Ethics*, **24**, 147–148.

Howe, K. R. (1987) Medical students' evaluation of different levels of medical ethics teaching: implications for curricula. *Medical Education*, **21**, 340–349.

Jacobson J. A., Tolle, S. W., Stocking, C., *et al* (1989) Internal medicine residents' preferences regarding medical ethics. *Academic Medicine*, **64**, 777–781.

Johnston, C. S. & Haughton, P. S. (2007) Teaching and learning ethics – medical students' perceptions of their ethics teaching. *Journal of Medical Ethics*, **33**, 418–422.

Kern, D. C., Parrino, T. A. & Korsai, D. R. (1985) The lasting value of clinical skills. *JAMA*, **254**, 72–76.

Loewy, E. H. (1986) Teaching medical ethics to medical students. *Journal of Medical Education*, **61**, 661–665.

Lynoe, N., Lofmark, R. & Thulesius, H. O. (2008) Teaching medical ethics: what is the impact of role models? Some experiences from Swedish medical schools. *Journal of Medical Ethics*, **34**, 315–316.

McDougall, R. (2009) Combating junior doctors' '4 a.m. logic': a challenge for medical ethics education. *Journal of Medical Ethics*, **35**, 203–206.

McElhinney, T. K. & Pellegrino, E. D. (1982) *The Humanities and Human Values in Medical Schools: A Ten Year Overview*. Society on Health and Human Values.

Miles, S. H., Lane, L. W., Bickel J., *et al* (1989) Medical ethics education: coming of age. *Academic Medicine*, **64**, 705–714.

Mitchell, K. R., Myser, C. & Kerridge, I. H. (1993) Assessing the clinical ethical competence of undergraduate medical students. *Journal of Medical Ethics*, **19**, 230–236.

Osborne, L. W. & Martin, C. W. (1989) The importance of listening to medical students' experiences when teaching them medical ethics. *Journal of Medical Ethics*, **15**, 35–38.

Patenaude, J., Niyonsenga, T. & Farard, D. (2003) Changes in students' moral development during medical school: a cohort study. *Canadian Medical Association Journal*, **168**, 840–844.

Rose, G. L. & Rukstalis, M. R. (2008) Imparting medical ethics: the role of mentorship in clinical training. *Mentoring and Tutoring: Partnership in Learning*, **16**, 77–89.

Rosenbaum, J. R., Bradley, E. H., Holmboe, E. S., *et al* (2004) Sources of ethical conflict in medical housestaff training: a qualitative study. *American Journal of Medicine*, **116**, 402–407.

Satterwhite, R. C., Satterwhite, W. M. & Enarson, C. (2000) An ethical paradox: the effect of unethical conduct on medical students' values. *Journal of Medical Ethics*, **26**, 462–465.

Savulescu, J., Crisp, R., Fulford, K. W., *et al* (1999) Evaluating ethics competence in medical education. *Journal of Medical Ethics*, **25**, 367–374.

Self, D. J., Wolinsky, F. D. & Baldwin, D. C. (1989) The effect of teaching medical ethics on medical students' moral reasoning. *Academic Medicine*, **64**, 755–759.

Self, D. J., Olivarez, M. & Baldwin, D. C. (1998) The amount of small-group case-study discussions needed to improve moral reasoning skills of medical students. *Academic Medicine*, **73**, 521–523.

Stirrat, G. M., Johnston, C., Gillon, R., *et al* on behalf of the Medical Education Working Group of the Institute of Medical Ethics and associated signatories (2010) Medical ethics and law for doctors of tomorrow: the 1998 Consensus Statement updated. *Journal of Medical Ethics*, **36**, 55–60.

Wong, J. G. W. S. & Cheung, E. P. T. (2003) Ethics assessment in medical students. *Medical Teacher*, **25**, 5–8.

CHAPTER 4

With the benefit of hindsight: lessons from history

Fiona Subotsky

Overview

This chapter looks first briefly at the medical codes and values of ancient Greece, and then those developing in the USA and the UK in the 19th century and beyond which help the understanding of today's approaches. Four well-documented historical cases of apparent medical boundary breaking are examined to see what was alleged or found, and how the doctors' contemporary colleagues, their patients and the public reacted. The cases are disparate and views may still differ as to the extent of the doctors' culpability, demonstrating both the frequent ambiguity of such situations, and how values and regulation have shifted over time.

Ancient Greece

The so-called Hippocratic oath of classical times, whether or not it was in widespread use, started with an invocation to the gods of medicine: Apollo the Olympian and the lesser demi-god Asclepius, with his daughters Hygieia and Panacea. It is usually not pointed out, however, that Apollo was a poor role model for doctors, being, like his father Zeus, a notorious womaniser, and tending to use force and deception to gain his ends. Indeed, he gave Cassandra, who refused his advances, the curse of never being believed. Such themes recur in more modern times.

The oath includes the following:

Into as many houses as I enter, I will go for the benefit of the ill, while being far from all voluntary and destructive injustice, especially from sexual acts both upon women's bodies and upon men's, both of the free and of slaves. (von Staden, 1996)

Miles (2004) comments that this is akin to the ancient Greek civil rules of hospitality which forbade a guest from having sexual relations with a member of the household against the wishes of the host. The action seemed to be viewed as a betrayal of trust of the householder, rather than the free or slave men, women and children in the house, who may or may not have been patients. The latter's lack of autonomy, or social and economic power, would have been reflected in difficulties in resistance or complaint. The presence of a specific prohibition indicates that the risk of such behaviour was recognised.

Aside from the injunctions in the oath there was discussion on how the outward show of good manners should correspond to inner moral virtue. This issue of 'medical decorum', or how a doctor should present himself, continued to be a topic for consideration and instruction through the centuries (Jonsen, 2000).

Early professionalisation

By the mid-19th century the American Medical Association had adopted a code of ethics (1847, revised 1903) based on the work of Percival, whose recommendations had been developed primarily to prevent in-fighting at the Manchester Royal Infirmary. The emphasis is somewhat curious to modern eyes, being largely about how physicians should behave towards each other, for instance not interfering with another doctor's treatment. Towards the patient, doctors are enjoined to 'unite tenderness, cheerfulness and firmness', to treat the patient with 'attention and humanity' and to take care to respect confidences. Actions should be such as to inspire hope and trust. For the benefit of public health, physicians should advise about such matters as vaccination and quarantine, oppose quacks and support pharmacists (American Medical Association, 1903).

Although rather vague, this was at least some guidance. The General Medical Council (GMC) of Great Britain and Ireland, established by the Medical Act of 1858, had a different approach. Its primary purpose was to establish a register of appropriately qualified doctors. It was empowered to erase a medical practitioner if, 'after due inquiry', a doctor was 'judged by the General Council to have been guilty of infamous conduct in any professional respect'. As a matter of policy, no guidance was given initially, nor were reasons given for decisions. Cases were judged one by one rather than by precedent. The two clearest indications were if the qualifying membership had been withdrawn, for instance by the Royal College of Surgeons (RCS), or if there had been a conviction for a serious offence, both of which relieved the GMC of directly determining culpability. For example, a Dr Morris was erased from the Medical Register in 1871 following his conviction for unlawful and indecent assault on the housekeeper of a patient (Smith, 1993). But why? Was it the conviction, the sexual element, or that the victim was a patient's servant? There is an echo of the wording of the Hippocratic oath in this decision. Membership of the RCS had also been withdrawn.

Eventually 'warning notices' were issued attached to the Medical Register, but the time lag on any given topic could be many years (Smith, 1993). The warning notice of 1920 gave advice under the formal headings of: 'Certificates, Notifications, Reports etc'; 'Unqualified Assistants and Covering'; 'Sale of Poisons'; 'Association with Unqualified Persons'; 'Advertising and Canvassing'; and 'Association with Women Practising as Midwives'. Essentially, these all concern trade restrictions. The Council also warned that other forms of professional misconduct were not excluded, 'as, for example, immorality involving abuse of professional relationship'. These strictures remained more or less identical for many years. In 1952, 'immorality' was replaced by 'adultery', whether as clarification or limitation is unclear. In 1960, the situation was elaborated: 'Any medical practitioner who abuses his professional position by committing adultery or improper conduct with a patient, or by maintaining an improper association with a patient, is liable to erasure' (General Medical Council, 1920, pp. viii–x; 1952, pp. viii–x; 1960, pp. ix–xi).

Reflecting on his years as Registrar, Draper (1983), noted that for many years there was an arrangement that 'all doctors found guilty of adultery in divorce proceedings in England were reported … to the Council' and investigated for abuse of the professional relationship. There was thus curiously active case finding, but a rather narrow view of what might constitute an improper sexual relationship. Spontaneous complainants, on the other hand, were usually put off by having to foot their own legal bills. Another deterrent would have been the full press reporting, as cases were heard in public.

Jean Robinson (1999) was involved with the GMC as chair of the Patients' Association and noted how slow the progress had been on the issue of reporting other colleagues for poor care or conduct. Indeed, this was thoroughly discouraged for many years; for instance, the 1981 *Fitness to Practise* guidance advised: 'The Council … regards as capable of amounting to serious professional misconduct … depreciation by a doctor of the professional skill, knowledge, qualification or service of another doctor' (General Medical Council, 1981, p. 14).

The situation in the UK and the USA is now greatly changed, with greater explicit demand for respect for the patient's autonomy, recognition of the doctor's position of power and consequent duty not to exploit vulnerability, awareness of potential conflicts of interest, and requirements to report poor practice. Nevertheless, scandals continue to occur, while doctors can be quite unaware of cases from the past, some of which are discussed next.

Sir William Wilde

This well-known and charismatic Dublin surgeon was brought to the public's attention with accusations of sexual misconduct in the course of practice (see Box 4.1). Previously his reputation as a ladies' man had been held rather to his credit. He probably hoped (largely correctly) that his general standing would protect him, especially as he had his wife's support. The public would have seen that his accuser's story was inconsistent: Was she chloroformed or suffocated? Was she raped or not? Why did she so frequently return after the alleged event? Why did she tell no one at the time? It would have seemed from her outrageous behaviour that she was a hysterical and unreliable girl, probably making accusations because of rejection and envy. It is not clear whether the seriousness of

---

Box 4.1 Sir William Wilde (1815–76), eminent surgeon

William Wilde was an extremely talented and successful eye and ear surgery pioneer in Dublin in the mid-19th century, with widespread international, social and literary contacts. He set up a hospital and dispensary for diseases of the eye and ear, and contributed largely to the effectiveness of the Irish census and its gathering of public health information. However, despite his knighthood in 1864, things began to turn sour.

His wife, Lady Wilde, was sued for libel by a Mary Travers for having complained to Mary's father about her behaviour. Mary, the daughter of another medical man, Professor Robert Travers, had originally consulted Sir William Wilde in 1854, aged 19. This developed into 'an acquaintanceship', according to him, or 'an intimacy' according to her. Anyway, they met regularly and openly for years, with William lending her small sums of money. Later, he gave larger sums for her to leave for Australia, which she did not.

According to Mary, in 1862, after William had examined a burn on her neck, he half-suffocated and then forced himself upon her while she was unconscious. She did, however, continue to visit.

In 1863 she published a pamphlet about a Dr Quilp (clearly William Wilde), who had chloroformed and raped a young lady. She distributed this widely, even picketing one of Wilde's lectures with placards advertising it. Lady Wilde was eventually spurred into action and wrote a letter of complaint to Mary's father. The ensuing libel trial was a focus of great interest as the extraordinary story unfolded. Wilde was formally co-defendant but did not take the stand, although at times the trial appeared to be more about his behaviour than his wife's alleged libel.

Lady Wilde, a famous and charismatic figure in her own right, known as the writer 'Speranza', appeared in court to be somewhat dismissive of the whole proceedings. It seems that she had found Mary quite a nuisance but had not at first especially attempted to stop the relationship. It was only when Mary began to make scenes in public that she reacted. The jury was somewhat baffled, found for Mary, but awarded only one farthing damages, leaving the Wildes to meet the considerable court costs.

Subsequently, nearly all the newspapers and medical journals supported Sir William and criticised Mary. His friends and colleagues rallied round with a series of social engagements, and he became professionally more in demand than ever. In 1865 Mary sued a newspaper which had said her story was unbelievable, and this time the jury decided against her. Nevertheless, Wilde's health deteriorated and he retreated somewhat from Dublin.

Sources: Hyde (1970); Wilson (1974); Melville (1994).

the allegation in the mind of the public related to the non-consensuality of the act, its adulterous nature, or violation of doctor–patient decorum. Maybe Mary Travers had to protect her own reputation, as an unmarried middle-class young woman, by saying that she was unconscious during the assault, whether by chloroform or by suffocation. This also served to reduce intrusive and embarrassing questioning at the trial, a situation which still prevents women coming forward with their experiences of sexual abuse.

This was all seen as highly entertaining by those attending court and the Dublin newspaper readers. Most of the medical press supported Wilde, as did his friends and colleagues, at least immediately after the trial. The GMC was not invoked (and would not at this stage have made any investigation without a conviction). It was not Wilde's registration but his reputation which was at stake and Mary Travers impugned this with some eventual success. What doctors contemplating a relationship with a patient might have learned was that it was an excellent idea to have powerful friends, a supportive wife and money for law suits. What patients might have learned was that the rules governing the doctor–patient relationship were extremely vague and that ignominy was certain to fall on any complainant, who would be regarded as hysterical if making a great deal of emotional fuss, or lying if she made little.

William Wilde's son Oscar might have benefited from considering the Travers case when instituting his own disastrous libel case – which ultimately led to his prison sentence (Ellmann, 1987, p. 15).

Isaac Baker Brown

This successful 19th-century surgeon was a pioneer in gynaecological technique, especially ovariectomy. His assertion that masturbation was the cause of much female nervous and hysterical dysfunction and advocacy of clitoridectomy as a cure-all led to campaigns by the *British Medical Journal* and the *Lancet* (see Box 4.2). The GMC does not feature in their discussions, but instead the Lunacy Commission was invoked. In the Obstetrical Society's debate on his expulsion, the grounds cited are important: lack of informed consent, from the patient, her family and friends and her personal doctor; 'quackery' – raising interest by advertising non-professionally; lack of logic to the approach; and lack of evidence of successful outcome. The lack of complaints was ascribed to shame. The specialist medical grouping was thought to hold the key to professional approval or otherwise, and was brought under pressure by the medical press.

Historical 'quackery' allegations are often viewed nowadays as a bid to stave off competition rather than to maintain a high quality of practice. It is fairer to assume both were relevant. What we do not have are any messages from the objects or victims of this extraordinary procedure, except for a large testimonial gift to Baker Brown from professional admirers and

Box 4.2 Isaac Baker Brown (1811–73), surgical gynaecologist

Isaac Baker Brown, from a modest but respectable background, became a member of the Royal College of Surgeons in 1834, and a Fellow in 1848. He practised in Connaught Square, London, and was a founder member of St Mary's Hospital. Baker Brown seized on the opportunities for the expansion of innovative surgery after the introduction of anaesthesia in 1847, soon becoming famous for his skill and daring in surgery for women. He was elected President of the Medical Society of London in 1865.

Although his first three ovariectomy patients died, Brown was so convinced of the efficacy that he operated next on his own sister. In 1848 he published *On Some Diseases of Women Admitting of Surgical Treatment*, but went further in 1866 with *The Curability of Certain Forms of Insanity, Epilepsy, Catalepsy and Hysteria in Females*. His theory was that many nervous conditions of women were due to masturbation, for which the cure would be the removal of the clitoris. He ensured his reputation for success was widespread, and cultivated rich socialites and the clergy for funds and referrals. He was not necessarily specific to patients and their families as to what was entailed. However, he operated openly, inviting other doctors in to see how he practised.

While it was thought at the time that much male insanity was due to masturbation, and cruel practices were designed to overcome it, in Britain (unlike in the USA and Europe), this had not been a widespread theory with respect to women. The *British Medical Journal* and the *Lancet* published articles condemning the approach and reported Baker Brown to the Lunacy Commission for operating on 'females of unsound mind' at his hospital, the London Surgical Home. The eminent 'alienists' of the day denied Baker Brown's claim to their support: Henry Maudsley (1866) wrote to say that in his experience female self-abuse was a consequence, not a cause of insanity; Forbes Winslow (1866) commented that 'Mr Baker Brown begins his treatment of these cases at the wrong end'.

After much dithering, a resolution of expulsion was brought before the Obstetrical Society of London. It was hotly debated, and fully reported in the *British Medical Journal*. Mr Seymour Haden described Baker Brown's publicity seeking and use of a baseless operation as a form of quackery; furthermore, the clitoridectomies were often performed without the full consent of the patient, her husband, or her medical attendant. Few dared to complain subsequently, as it would seem to be an admission of immoral practice. Baker Brown was found against; his practice quickly fell off and his health severely deteriorated. After his death, his apparent failure of judgement was put down to a post-mortem finding of very extensive cerebral softening.

Sources: Dally (1991, pp. 147–184); Black (1997); Roy (2004).

grateful patients comprising a six-piece silver dessert service valued at 300 guineas.

Clitoridectomy fell out of fashion in Britain, but not in the USA, and ovariectomy continued, often for similar 'nervous problems'. The ground rules for professional practice were made no clearer (Dally, 1991, pp. 147–184; Darby, 2007).

Ernest Jones

Ernest Jones' own account, and most of his biographies, understandably rather gloss over the episodes recounted in Box 4.3, but more recently greater attention has been paid to the likelihood of the repeated concerns having some substance. The case of the schoolchildren is instructive:

Box 4.3 Ernest Jones (1879–1958), Freud's collaborator and biographer

After gaining brilliant academic qualifications, Ernest Jones became resident medical officer at the North-Eastern Hospital for Children in London in 1903. Having fallen out with the matron, he was forced to resign – ostensibly for taking absence without leave. Subsequently, despite multiple applications, he never gained a substantive hospital clinical appointment in Britain, but had a variety of part-time appointments.

By 1906 he was working in a part-time post for the Education Department of the London County Council (LCC), with responsibilities in mental deficiency schools. One afternoon was spent assessing a number of children for their speech development, following which four children, a boy and three girls aged 12–14 years, complained to the headmistress about the doctor's behaviour. She reported the matter, and Dr Kerr, the LCC Medical Officer for Education, interviewed the girls with Jones present. Dr Kerr concluded that the girls must have made it up between them. Nevertheless, one of the girl's parents took the matter to the police. Further questioning of the girls and analysis of stains on a tablecloth led to Jones' arrest. Detailed reports of the subsequent hearings do not exist, but the girls' accounts were disbelieved, with laughter in court, while Jones did not take the stand. The newspapers and medical journals rejoiced, and a party was held at the house of Sir Victor Horsley, President of the Royal College of Surgeons of England, where funds raised to pay for the legal costs were formally presented to Jones.

In 1908, Jones was again asked to resign from a hospital post, where he was formally a pathologist, for examining two female patients without a chaperone, and asking 'certain questions' of one girl, aged 10, whose parents complained. Jones' own later account was that the girl had a hysterical paralysis whose sexual origin he was able to determine by his questioning.

He left for Canada, where rumours of inappropriately sexualised treatment continued, such as recommending masturbation or going to prostitutes, and showing his patients obscene postcards. One patient accused him of having had sexual intercourse with her and threatened to shoot him. While he described her as 'a severe hysteric' and 'pronouncedly homosexual', nevertheless he gave her $500 to prevent further scandal. In 1910 Jones had told Freud: 'Now I have always been conscious of sexual attractions to patients; my wife was a patient of mine.'

Ernest Jones' later career within the psychoanalytic movement was an eminent one. Much depended on by Sigmund Freud, he founded the British Psycho-Analytical Society and was Freud's official biographer, edited his works and helped many Jewish analysts, including Freud, escape from Nazi persecution.

Sources: Gabbard (2002); Kuhn (2002); Maddox (2006).

---

clearly the headmistress believed them and the police took their evidence seriously. Reconstruction of their allegations is difficult as details are not recorded, presumably because of their 'delicacy'. For instance, the nature of the tablecloth stain was discussed only when ladies had withdrawn from the court. Meanwhile, the stories of the girls were discredited – after all, they were young, female and mentally limited. For the court, their evidence was outweighed by the standing of a respectable medical man with peer support. It appears that a matron, a headmistress and parents were the most concerned, while medical colleagues resisted suggestions of guilt. Yet even within the medical world the lack of job offers despite excellent qualifications suggests that there may have been a word-of-mouth notification system. There is no mention of a GMC referral, which anyway would have been unlikely to have proceeded without a conviction. Even now, resort to private practice and leaving the country recur as responses to allegations of sexual misconduct.

When Jones first became involved with psychoanalysis, major tenets included: that the hysterical patient's reports of early sexual trauma were fantasies; that neurosis could follow from the repression of sexual desire; and that patients were likely to fall in love with their analysts (the transference effect). None of these would have checked any aberrant tendencies in the analyst. While Freud himself counselled against sexual involvement with patients, many others in the early psychoanalytic movement took little heed of this advice. What would now be regarded as extraordinary boundary breaking was commonplace. Gabbard (2002), commenting on this situation, notes that colleagues (unless female) typically sided with the analyst complained against, and suggests that both misogyny and secret admiration were at play.

Heinrich Gross

During the Second World War, Heinrich Gross (see Box 4.4) was one of many doctors involved in the Nazi killing programme which was intended to improve the German race and release resources for the fit. Doctors, and especially psychiatrists, had been prime movers in the eugenicist movement, which had started with compulsory sterilisation of those who were mentally ill or handicapped. This latter activity was internationally widespread, and Germans were able to claim accurately that the Americans had led the way. Why and how could this happen? The motives of the German doctors studied seem often to have been ambition, research interest and support of nationalist moral values, as much as fear or sadistic psychopathology. Senior academics were eager to have both live and dead human material to study and experiment on. There were few serious reprisals for refusal. Paths for acceptance were made easy and rewarding. Each step could be small and routinised, and therefore more easily distanced from the whole.

Box 4.4 Heinrich Gross (1915–2005), Austrian child psychiatrist

During the Second World War Heinrich Gross was one of the head doctors at Am Spiegelgrund, the children's section of Vienna's large mental hospital, Am Steinhof. In 1938 Austria had been incorporated into Nazi Germany and its medical system took up the 'T4' programme – a eugenic mission, beyond sterilisation, to terminate 'life unworthy of life'. Falling into this category were people who were mentally ill or mentally handicapped, especially if already in institutions; later, any misfit of race or behaviour was included. The development of the gas killing systems was for this purpose.

The killing of children was more subtle, and special training was provided. First, children were notified as possibly qualifying 'cases'. After refereeing of the forms, those deemed suitable were sent to special paediatric hospitals for 'treatment', often far from home. They were put on starvation diets, given sedatives orally and by injection, subjected to painful and risky experiments and exposed to cold. Over 700 children died in this way at Spiegelgrund, with Gross's signature on 238 of the children's death certificates. One of Gross's patients who survived described him coming to the wards to select children – first 'the bedwetters, or harelips or the slow thinkers.... We did not dare ask where they were taken. We never saw them again.' Gross saw the opportunity for personal scientific advancement in collecting interesting specimens and making painful investigations, such as pneumo-encephalography, without medical indication.

Gross was not available for the Nuremberg trials as he was being held by the Russians, though the chief of Am Spiegelgrund, Dr Illing, was executed. Gross was charged three times in Austria. The first trial resulted in a conviction for manslaughter and was overturned on a technicality. The second was abandoned because of a statute of limitations. The third trial was suspended on the ground of his advanced age and alleged dementia. Meanwhile, he had returned to Am Steinhof and made his name as a forensic expert, also publishing results of research on the remains of the child victims, boasting that his brain collection was the finest in the world. The child victims' brains were held for decades in the hospital, and buried finally in 2002.

Dr Gross died a free man at the age of 90.

Sources: Müller-Hill (1998); Thomas *et al* (2006).

The programme was identified as a medical one, even to the requirement to have a doctor turn on the tap for the gassing chambers (Lifton, 1986; Annas & Grodin, 1992).

Protests become more vocal by 1941, led by the Catholic Church rather than medical organisations, and the systematic euthanasia programme was called to a halt. However, this meant that the gas chamber equipment and expertise, having largely fulfilled its task of emptying the asylums, was moved to use for exterminating the inmates of concentration camps. Meanwhile, within the asylums, non-systematic killing continued, now described as the period of 'wild euthanasia'. Such was the case at Spiegelgrund.

After the war, there were trials of many doctors. The proceedings concentrated on their abandonment of ethical approaches for the good of patients in favour of 'research'. The outcome was the development of the Nuremberg code, which stresses the importance of informed consent (Weindling, 2004). Important as this was, by concentrating on the 'research' aspects, it was as if the grotesque evil of the whole underpinning medical system could hardly be faced. This also allowed the outside world to think that their own doctors must be different, and seemingly allowed many compliant Nazi doctors themselves to continue to think that they had done a good job in difficult circumstances.

Conclusion

While the Hippocratic precepts clearly require the intention of benefit and interdict injustice, such medical ethics as were discussed in the 19th and early 20th centuries tended to focus on pleasant manners and good relationships between doctors. Regulation was very limited. Conflicts of interest, for instance between the individual and state, or between research and clinical values, were little articulated. While the criminal justice system, medical peer group and press could provide formal or informal sanction, they were of little correctional value if controlled by the state, as in the Third Reich.

The four doctors instanced worked across Europe over a wide time period. While varying considerably in their actions, they clearly abused their professional positions to take advantage of patients. Their vices were not of ignorance or neglect; indeed, each had outstanding qualities. None regretted the activities of which he was accused, although two (Wilde and Baker Brown), having been eminent and successful clinicians, suffered in their health and withdrew after negative judgements. The other two (Jones and Gross) each survived a series of accusations and went on to have extremely successful careers. The voices of the patients were rarely heard. The victims, who were often female, children and/or mentally ill, had little autonomy and were rarely believed. Criticism from other doctors was often absent and the achievement of eminence was no bar to the possibility of the abuse of medical power. All this is still relevant today.

References

American Medical Association (1903) *Principles of Medical Ethics*. Online at http://www.ama-assn.org/ama1/pub/upload/mm/43/1903principalsofethi.pdf (accessed 17 June 2009).

Annas, G. J. & Grodin, M. A. (1992) *The Nazi Doctors and the Nuremberg Code: Human Rights in Human Experimentation*. Oxford University Press.

Black, J. (1997) Female genital mutilation: a contemporary issue, and a Victorian obsession. *Journal of the Royal Society of Medicine*, **90**, 402–406.

Dally, A. (1991) *Women Under the Knife: A History of Surgery*. Hutchinson Radius.

Darby, R. (2007) The benefits of psychological surgery: John Scoffern's satire on Isaac Baker Brown. *Medical History*, **51**, 527–544.

Draper, M.R. (1983) The GMC from 1950 to 1982: a Registrar's impression. In *GMC Annual Report for 1982*, pp. 11–20. General Medical Council.

Ellmann, R. (1988) *Oscar Wilde*. Penguin Books.

Gabbard, G. O. (2002) Boundary violations and the abuse of power: commentary on paper by Philip Kuhn. *Studies in Gender and Sexuality*, **3**, 379–388.

General Medical Council (1920) *Medical Register*, pp. viii–x. London: General Medical Council.

General Medical Council (1952) *Medical Register*, pp. viii–x. GMC.

General Medical Council (1960) *Medical Register*, pp ix–xi. GMC.

General Medical Council (1981) *Professional Conduct and Discipline: Fitness to Practise*. GMC.

Hyde. H. M. (1970) *Their Good Names: Twelve Cases of Libel and Slander with some Introductory Reflections on the Law*. Hamish Hamilton.

Jonsen, A. R. (2000) *A Short History of Medical Ethics*, pp. 7–8. Oxford University Press.

Kuhn, P. (2002) 'Romancing with a wealth of detail': narratives of Ernest Jones' 1906 trial for indecent assault. *Studies in Gender and Sexuality*, **3**, 344–378.

Lifton, R. J. (1986) *The Nazi Doctors: Medical Killing and the Psychology of Genocide*. Basic Books.

Maddox, B. (2006) *Freud's Wizard: The Enigma of Ernest Jones*. John Murray.

Maudsley, H. (1866) Clitoridectomy (letter). *British Medical Journal*, ii, 705.

Melville, J. (1994) *Mother of Oscar: The Life of Francesca Jane Wilde*. John Murray.

Miles, S. H. (2004) *The Hippocratic Oath and the Ethics of Medicine*. Oxford University Press.

Müller-Hill, Benno (1998) *Murderous Science: Elimination by Scientific Selection of Jews, Gypsies and Others in Germany, 1933–1945* (trans. G. R. Fraser). Cold Spring Harbor Laboratory Press:

Robinson, J. (1999) The price of deceit: the reflections of an advocate. In *Medical Mishaps: Pieces of the Puzzle* (eds M. M. Rosenthal, L. Mulcahy & S. Lloyd-Bostock), pp. 246–256. Open University Press.

Roy, J. M. (2004) Brown, Isaac Baker (1811–1873). *Oxford Dictionary of National Biography*. Oxford University Press. Online at http://oxforddnb.com/view article/50268 (accessed 22 April 2009).

Smith, R. G. (1993) The development of ethical guidance for medical practitioners by the General Medical Council. *Medical History*, **37**, 6–67.

Thomas, F. P., Beres, A. & Shevell, M. (2006) 'A cold wind coming': Heinrich Gross and child euthanasia in Vienna. *Journal of Child Neurology*, **21**, 342–348.

von Staden, H. (1996) 'In a pure and holy way': personal and professional conduct in the Hippocratic oath. *Journal of the History of Medicine and Allied Sciences*, **51**, 406–408.

Weindling, P. J. (2004) *Nazi Medicine and the Nuremberg Trials: From Medical War Crimes to Informed Consent*. Palgrave Macmillan.

Wilson, T. G. (1974) *Victorian Doctor: Being the Life of Sir William Wilde*. EP Publishing.

Winslow, F. (1866) Clitoridectomy (letter). *British Medical Journal*, ii, 706.

CHAPTER 5

The prevalence of boundary violations between mental health professionals and their clients

Tanya Garrett

Overview

Boundary violation by professionals, especially sexual, has been of academic and media interest in recent years, and there have been some high-profile cases of professionals being criticised and punished for abusing their position. 'Dual role' relationships are also a concern, for instance financial involvement with clients. Nevertheless, there is little coordinated, consistent information or research available in the UK regarding the prevalence of abuse of clients by professionals. This chapter examines the methodological difficulties, available studies and what types of abuse and boundary violation have been covered.

Introduction

Estimating the prevalence of boundary violations between mental health professionals and their clients is very difficult. Most research in this area has focused on abuse (rather than boundary violations *per se*) of clients by professionals, in particular sexual abuse. Public concern in the UK has been heightened by a number of recent well publicised cases of, and inquiries into, sexual abuse of clients within the National Health Service (NHS), such as the cases of Clifford Ayling (see Box 10.1, p. 115), and Michael Haslam (see Box 6.1, p. 65) and William Kerr (see Box 6.2, p. 66) (Paufley, 2004; Department of Health, 2005). There has been little attention afforded to other forms of abuse, such as emotional or physical abuse, and even less to other types of boundary violations, such as financial gain.

There are various sources of data regarding sexual contact between professionals and clients, but the combination of little research and lack of detail in recording procedures results in an extremely unclear picture in respect of the phenomenon of professional–client boundary violation in the British healthcare system. There is also an important issue in relation to under-reporting, with clients, staff and relatives feeling unable to initiate or pursue complaints (Donaldson, 1994).

The available research data, largely from other countries, despite their methodological limitations (see below), suggest that approximately 7% of mental health professionals violate the sexual boundary in therapy and a variety of types of sexual contact occur, with such abuse beginning both during therapy and after discharge. A similar percentage appear to violate the financial boundary. A far greater proportion form social relationships with current or ex-clients and have non-sexual physical contact with them. The prevalence of emotional abuse of clients is impossible to estimate due to lack of research in this regard worldwide, but in the UK information from Witness, a professional boundaries charity (formerly Prevention of Professional Abuse Network, POPAN), suggests that it is not insignificant.

Definitions

In this chapter, the terms 'therapist' and 'professional' are used interchangeably to refer to mental health workers, and should be taken to refer equally to all those who treat clients or patients within the British mental health system. Similarly, the term 'therapy' is used to refer to professional contact between mental health professionals and their clients in a generic sense.

Sexual contact with clients includes kissing, genital exposure, touching the breasts, fondling the genital area, oral sex and sexual intercourse (vaginal and anal). All these forms are regarded by most authorities as abusive and are almost universally considered a serious boundary violation between professional and client. Touching and hugging are less clear-cut and may not always include a sexual component (Jehu, 1994).

Methodological difficulties

Research may be flawed due to factors such as sampling bias in terms of the motivation of those mailed in surveys to participate or not: it might be argued that response and disclosure rates could be biased either by increased response from therapists who perceive their sexual contact with clients as having exerted a harmful effect or, alternatively, by those who view such contact in positive terms.

In addition, the demographic characteristics of therapists who have sexual contact with their clients, particularly in relation to returning questionnaires, are unknown. Thus it is problematic to draw inferences about the larger population of such therapists on the basis of such studies (Williams, 1992). In surveys, respondents may be prevented from responding at all, or from responding honestly, due to fear of lack of anonymity or confidentiality, even when these are assured by the researcher. The characteristics of those who do not respond to surveys are unknown. Further, it is not clear how many of those who do respond but who claim to have had no sexual contact with clients are in fact presenting a false picture. It is important to note that those surveys which offer a definition of sexual contact may inadvertently exclude some forms of therapist–client sexual contact, thus restricting 'case' reporting. Most researchers have included a definition of sexual contact in their surveys, which may limit the range of sexual acts which respondents describe.

It is difficult to draw inferences about changes in therapists' sexual behaviour with their clients over time, because surveys do not specify when the sexual behaviour occurred (Williams, 1992). The information gained may also depend on whether post-termination sexual contacts are included in the figures. Most studies have not provided their respondents with specific instructions as to whether to include or exclude sexual contacts with clients where the client was discharged when the sexual liaison began. Reporting practices, particularly by male psychotherapists, may have changed over recent years (Stake & Oliver, 1991) because of the increased publicity which has been accorded to the sanctions applicable to sexually abusive professionals. Thus, Schoener (1991) concluded that there is no evidence to suggest that a decline is taking place in the incidence or prevalence of therapist–client sexual contact.

Types of boundary violations

Grunebaum (1986) described information from a survey of clients who reported that they were harmed by therapy. The most common cause of such harm was the client feeling that the relationship with the therapist was distant and rigid. Emotional seductiveness, sexual abuse, multiple involvement in therapy cults and a poor match between therapist and client were also noted. Mogul (1992) noted that most ethics complaints against female psychiatrists in the USA concerned sexual misconduct. There were also complaints involving discourtesy or poor judgement, breach of confidentiality, and financial matters (usually billing disputes).

Financial issues

Over 6% of respondents in a study by Borys & Pope (1989) had accepted a gift worth over $50 from a client, 0.2% had borrowed over $20 from a client, and over 20% reported that they had purchased goods or services from a client. However, the latest guidelines from the American Psychological Association (2003) reversed its long-standing policy on barter and now allow it on a limited basis.

Social contact

In Borys & Pope's (1989) study, over 30% of participants had established a friendship with a client after termination of treatment, and 11.5% had eaten in a restaurant with a client after a session. Over 7% had invited clients to a personal party or social event, over 10% had provided therapy to an employee, and over 10% had provided therapy to someone who was at the time a student or supervisee. Over 7% had employed a client, and almost 29% had disclosed details of current personal stresses.

The use of touch

It is clear from research that if touch is used at all in therapy, it should be employed judiciously and with caution (Edwards, 1981), as it can be extremely damaging for clients, for example those who have been sexually abused as children. More damaged clients can experience a loss of inhibition if touched, or can see touch by a professional as a sexual promise, which, when unfulfilled, can be seen as betrayal or abandonment. Further, there can be a link between therapists (particularly male) touching their clients and engaging in sexual contact (Kardener *et al*, 1976; Holroyd & Brodsky, 1980). Thus, the decision to touch or not to touch clients must include a consideration of the client's possible perceptions, and interpretations of the touch, and the therapist's motivations for using it (Holub & Lee, 1990). There are many different types of touch, from nurturing to aggressive, from prompting to sexual. The use of some of these types of touch may be more problematic than others.

Perhaps in response to such considerations, the American Psychological Association (1982, cited in Goodman & Teicher, 1988, p. 492) adopted the following statement regarding physical contact with clients: 'permissible physical touching is defined as that conduct which is based upon the exercise of professional judgment, and which, implicitly, comports with accepted standards of professional conduct'. This careful wording would appear to be supported by the research, although perhaps not always followed in practice.

The use of physical contact with clients is a relatively common practice in psychotherapy. Results of a survey by Pope *et al* (1987) showed that a quarter of psychologist respondents had kissed a client, 44.5% hugged clients rarely, and 41.7% did so more frequently (i.e. a total of 86.2% of respondents had hugged a client at some point in their career). Most were prepared to shake their client's hand and did not consider this unethical. Holroyd & Brodsky (1977) found that 27% of their respondents engaged in non-erotic physical contact, mostly humanistically oriented therapists. Among general physicians, more female practitioners than male believe in, and use, non-erotic touch (Perry, 1976). Unpublished data from the

International Study of the Development of Psychotherapists (J. Davis, 1995, personal communication) show that 54.8% of a sample of psychotherapists engaged in non-sexual physical contact other than a handshake with their clients. What clients recall is unknown, however, and this is certainly an area which would benefit from further research.

In the light of these potential concerns, therapists should think carefully about touching their clients. Kertay & Reviere (1993) advocate a three-level approach regarding decision-making in this area. First, the issue of ethical violations should be considered: those therapists who recognise that they are likely to touch clients selectively on the basis of the client's gender should avoid the use of touch. When touch leads to sexual arousal on the part of either therapist or client, it should be discontinued. The second level of decision-making relates to the 'necessary qualities' of the therapeutic relationship. Various aspects of the therapeutic relationship should be considered: touch should not be employed in the early stages of therapy; and it must be congruent to the relationship between the client and the therapist, and to the needs of the client. Finally, the therapist and client should discuss the use of touch and, in particular, potential sexual feelings which may arise. This approach assumes that the therapist is motivated to behave ethically and to take steps to avoid sexual contact with clients, which, of course, applies to some, but not all, therapists.

Emotional abuse

Emotional abuse was the most common type of abuse reported to POPAN by clients, but was also often a precursor to other types of abuse, which included physical, financial, racial and sexual abuse (Blunden & Nash, undated a,b). In a sample of 240 cases referred to POPAN over 9 months in 1998, it was found that 69% involved emotional abuse, 42% sexual abuse, 8% physical abuse, and 4% each financial and racial abuse.

Sexual boundary violations

Williams (1992) suggests that multiple sources of information should be used when attempting to establish the prevalence of sexual contact between professionals and their clients, including surveys of professionals and clients, as well as data from courts and professional ethics bodies. Each source has its limitations. For example, it is likely that professionals may be unwilling to report their own unethical behaviour even anonymously. Thus, survey data are likely to underestimate sexual contact between professionals and clients. Clients may also under-report, for a variety of reasons, such as shame and fear (Donaldson, 1994). Data from professional organisations and the courts may be imperfect because 'only serious violations are likely to be reported' (Sarkar, 2004). Certainly, from the author's experience as a member of the Investigatory Committee of the British Psychological Society (which until recently screened all complaints), it is sometimes difficult to progress a complaint of sexual misconduct where the complainant, as is often the case, is reluctant to make a complaint to the police, and where there is likely to be little or no evidence other than the two individuals' accounts. It is also possible that false accusations can confound the picture.

Information from surveys of professionals

Most research in this area has been undertaken in the USA. It has not revealed differences in the prevalence of sexual contact with clients between the main statutory psychotherapy professions of psychology, psychiatry and social work (Borys & Pope, 1989). No information is as yet available to indicate the extent of sexual contact between other professionals, lay psychotherapists and counsellors, and their clients.

On the whole, it has been reported in US studies that under 10% of professional psychotherapists have had sexual contact with their clients. Quadrio (1996) estimates a similar prevalence rate among psychiatrists in Australia, based on cases prosecuted in New South Wales. In the UK, Garrett & Davies (1998) report that 3.4% of their national sample of clinical psychologists described engaging in what they considered to be sexual contact with their clients. A survey of 850 senior NHS medical staff carried out in northern England reported that, over a 5-year period, serious concerns were raised about 6% of the senior medical staff (Donaldson, 1994). Of these 49 cases, seven related to 'sexual matters', defined as 'sexual overtones in dealing with clients, or staff, or both'. Complaints were made initially by clients, relatives or staff. All but one of the medical staff in this category took early retirement after the complaint.

Kardener *et al* (1973), in their study of US psychiatrists, indicate a prevalence of 6–7% for all forms of 'erotic contact'. Pope *et al* (1979), also in a study of US psychiatrists, found that 7% admitted to sexual contact (a term that was undefined) with clients. Derosis *et al* (1987) found that 6.6% of the psychiatrist respondents in their North American survey had engaged in 'sexual contact' with their clients, although again the term was not defined. Similarly, Gartrell *et al* (1986) identify a figure of 6.4% of North American psychiatrists who reported engaging in 'contact which was intended to arouse or satisfy sexual desire in the patient, therapist, or both'.

Holroyd & Brodsky (1980) found that 3.2% of North American psychologist respondents to their survey had had sexual intercourse with a client, and another 4.6% engaged in other types of sexual behaviour (total 7.8%). In another survey of psychologists conducted in the USA, Pope *et al* (1986) report a rate of 6.5% for 'sexual intimacies' on the part of psychologists with clients, although the researchers do not give the original wording of the question, or define sexual intimacy. In Pope *et al*'s subsequent (1987)

Table 5.1 Proportions of professionals reporting sexual contact with clients

Profession	Source	Country	Percentage
Psychiatrists	Kardener *et al* (1973)	USA	6–7
	Pope *et al* (1979)	USA	7
	Derosis *et al* (1987)	USA	6.6
	Gartrell *et al* (1987)	USA	6.4
Psychologists	Holroyd & Brodsky (1980)	USA	7.8
	Pope *et al* (1986)	USA	6.5
	Pope *et al* (1987)	USA	1.9
	Pope & Tabachnick (1993)	USA	9.4
	Rodolfa *et al* (1994)	USA	4
	Garrett & Davis (1998)	UK	3.4
Social workers	Gechtman (1989)	USA	3.8
	Bernsen *et al* (1994)	USA	2.2
Counsellors	Thoreson *et al* (1993)	USA	8.7
Marriage/family counsellors	Boatwright (1989, cited in Sonne & Pope, 1991)	USA	13

study of psychologists, only 1.9% reported having 'engaged in erotic activity with a client'. Pope & Tabachnick (1993) mailed a questionnaire to 'applied' psychologist members of the American Psychological Association. Twenty-seven therapists (10 women and 17 men) (9.4%) were identified as experiencing 'sexual involvement' in therapy, defined as such by themselves. Rodolfa *et al* (1994) report a rate of 4% of psychologists, again in the USA, who admitted to 'sexual intimacies' with clients, and then only 'rarely'.

In a study of social workers in the USA, Gechtman (1989) found that 3.8% of respondents reported having 'erotic' contact with clients. Bernsen *et al* (1994) found that 3.6% of male and 0.5% of female social workers surveyed practising in the USA (overall 2.2%) reported 'sex with a client'. Although Thoreson *et al* (1993) found that only 1.7% of their sample of US male counsellors reported sexual intercourse or direct genital stimulation with current clients, a further 7% reported such contact with discharged clients. Presumably the figures would have been higher had a broader definition of sexual contact been adopted.

The surveys are summarised in Table 5.1.

From the available information, sexual acts which take place between therapists and their clients include: suggestive behaviour, clients stripping to underwear, being naked above (female only) or below the waist, telling a sexual fantasy to a client, erotic kissing, therapists lying on top of or underneath a client, touching, fondling, massage, genital exposure, masturbation, oral–genital contact, hand–genital contact, anal intercourse and vaginal intercourse (Bouhoutsos *et al*, 1983; Vinson, 1987; D'Addario, 1977, cited in Pope & Bouhoutsos, 1986; Gartrell *et al*, 1986; Kuchan, 1989; Valiquette, 1989, cited in Jehu, 1994; Pope & Tabachnick, 1993).

Sexual intercourse occurs in anything between 41% (Holroyd & Brodsky, 1980) and 83% (D'Addario, 1977, cited in Pope & Bouhoutsos, 1986) of cases where sexual contact has taken place, with other studies suggesting figures somewhere in between, for example 58% (Bouhoutsos 1985) and 75% (Vinson, 1987).

Around 18% of sexual contacts taking place during therapy occur in sessions and 17% concurrent with therapy but outside therapy sessions (Gartrell *et al*, 1986). The remainder occur after termination of therapy (see below).

Recurrent sexual contact

From the limited evidence available there appears to be some discrepancy in the proportions of therapists reported to have had sexual relations with more than one client. It is important to note the finding that therapists who have sexual contact with one client are at a high risk of repeating this behaviour (Gartrell *et al*, 1986). In a study of psychiatrists, 33% of those who admitted having a sexual relationship had done so with more than one client (Gartrell *et al*, 1986). The number of clients abused by a single therapist ranged up to 12. Quadrio (1996) also reports that one-third of the abusive therapists described by the clients in her study were 'repeat offenders'. Earlier studies suggest higher figures: Holroyd & Brodsky (1977) found that 80% of the clinical psychologists who had had sexual contact with clients in their study had done so with more than one client, and one therapist had victimised 10. Such figures would accord with the 75% of psychiatrists who reported sexual contact who also stated that they had been sexually involved with more than one client (Butler & Zelen, 1977).

Sexual intimacy with ex-clients

Sexual intimacy with discharged clients is rarely mentioned in the literature, and many of the epidemiological surveys do not differentiate between current and discharged clients. Yet it is important because it has been argued that sexual contact with discharged clients may be acceptable, despite the evidence which suggests that it may be just as damaging for the client as sexual contact while in therapy. In a study which did draw a distinction between current and former clients, 29.6% of psychiatrists surveyed stated that they believed that post-termination sexual contact with clients would sometimes be acceptable (Gartrell *et al*, 1987). Interestingly, 74% of the psychiatrists in this study who had had sexual contact with clients believed that such contact would be acceptable, and indeed used this as a means of rationalising their behaviour. Indeed, it is possible that therapists may terminate treatment *in order* to engage in sexual contact (Coleman, 1988). In around three-quarters of cases, therapists began a sexual relationship with their clients after termination of therapy. Figures vary from 69% (Gartrell *et al*, 1986) to 77% (Pope & Vetter, 1991).

Duration of the contact

In one of the few studies to address the question of the duration of therapist–client sexual contact, Gartrell *et al* (1986) report the length of therapist–client sexual 'relationships' as between one sexual encounter (19%) and over 5 years (17%), with other categories as follows: less than 3 months, 26%; 3–11 months, 17%; 1–5 years, 21%. Garrett & Davis (1998) used the same categories and found that, of those respondents who reported the duration of their sexual contact, 44% reported once-only encounters; less than 3 months, 22%; 3–11 months, 11%; and 22% had endured for more than 5 years. The largest group of therapists and clients were sexually involved for a relatively short period – less than 3 months (Gartrell *et al* in the US) and one-off encounters (Garrett & Davis in the UK).

Information from insurance companies

Approximately 13% of allegations of professional misconduct handled by the American Psychological Association insurance trust in 1981 and 18% of the complaints to the American Psychological Association ethics committee in 1982 involved sexual 'offences' against clients. Yet suits and complaints were rarely filed, in only about 4% of cases, and only half of these were completed (Bouhoutsos, 1985).

In the UK, the Medical Protection Society collects information regarding criminal convictions against registered medical practitioners, but this is not available on their website. The Medical Defence Union does not publish relevant data and its database is not amenable to a search for such information. Similarly, insurance bodies providing cover to other professionals do not provide information on their websites regarding claims made.

Information from professional bodies/state licensing boards, regulators and charities

Little information is available from the USA regarding the activities of US state licensing boards. However, Gottlieb *et al* (1988) found that over a period of 3 years (1982–85), the total number of complaints against psychologists of sexual impropriety within therapeutic relationships rose dramatically, by over 480%. In a survey of the records of a large US state's psychology licensing and disciplinary board over 28 months, Pope (1993) found 22 cases in which sexual contact with a client led to the therapist being disciplined. In North America at least, there have been approximately three times more malpractice cases involving psychiatrists than those involving psychologists (Perr, 1989), though this finding may be accounted for by the larger number of psychiatrists in practice.

Table 5.2 Professions of alleged abusers

Profession	1 April 1998– 31 December 1998[a]	1998–99[a]
Doctors	25% (60)	27% (psychiatrists, 9%; general practitioners, 17%; other, 2%)
Psychotherapists	25% (60)	24%
Counsellors	14% (31)	11%
Nurses	10% (23)	11%
Psychologists	7% (16)	7%
Social workers	4% (9)	4%
Osteopaths	–	2%
Clergy	–	4%
Others (including unregistered care workers, support staff and volunteers)	–	6%

[a] April–December 1998 column gives percentages followed by actual numbers in parentheses; 1998–99 column gives percentages only, as actual numbers not available.
Source: POPAN.

Although the nature of complaints is not specified, it is possible to search the GMC's website for information regarding individual decisions on fitness to practise. Sarkar (2004) noted that the GMC no longer published details of the types of case that came before its Professional Conduct Committee, but in the past approximately six cases of sexual misconduct were heard by the GMC each year, and of these about three resulted in a finding against the practitioner.

POPAN/Witness has published some information regarding its activity (Blunden & Nash, undated *a*), although the nature of this information is varied and often numbers are not available. Consistent data for each year are not available, so these data should be viewed with caution. However, the available information is given in Table 5.2.

The number of individuals contacting POPAN has increased annually (Blunden & Nash, undated *a*). In 1998–99, there were a total of 637 'cases', which included 394 individual new enquiries, 20 cases offered advocacy and support, 58 information-and-support cases, 61 existing enquiries, and 104 individuals offered continuing support.

Information from surveys of clients/client sources

Few surveys of clients have been conducted in relation to sexual contact with therapists; most of the little research in this area is of a qualitative nature, and has not addressed the issue of prevalence. A psychology clinic in California that advertised (presumably locally) for potential recruits to a group therapy programme for clients who had been sexually intimate with a therapist received 25 responses (Sonne *et al*, 1985). Two researchers have recruited clients reporting sexual abuse by a therapist for research purposes (Russell, 1993; Quadrio, 1996), but these were not formal surveys. Each of these researchers interviewed 40 such clients. In a survey of therapy clients who were also clinical psychologists, Pope & Feldman-Summers (1992) found that almost 7% had been sexually involved with their therapists. In a study of psychologists who had treated clients who had been sexually involved with a previous therapist, Pope & Vetter (1991) found that only 12% of the clients had filed complaints.

There have been no national surveys of clients undertaken in the UK. However, Garrett & Davis (1998) found that just under 23% of a sample of over 500 UK clinical psychologists had treated clients who reported having been sexually intimate with previous therapists.

Future directions

It is clear that further research is required in the area of abuse of clients and boundary violations in general. In the UK especially there has been poor collection and dissemination of regulatory or complaints data, and there has been little research into prevalence, irrespective of methodological difficulties. Systematic UK data regarding the client experience is also sadly lacking.

References

American Psychological Association (2003) *Ethical Principles of Psychologists and Code of Conduct*. American Psychological Association.

Bernsen, A., Tabachnick, B. G. & Pope, K. S. (1994) National survey of social workers' sexual attraction to their clients: results, implications, and comparison to psychologists. *Ethics and Behavior*, **4**, 369–388.

Blunden, F. & Nash, J. (undated *a*) Tackling abuse of patients and clients – the work of POPAN. Unpublished article. Online at http://www.popan.org.uk. (Accessed January 2010.)

Blunden, F. & Nash, J. (undated *b*) The prevention of client abuse in psychotherapy. Unpublished article. Online at http://www.popan.org.uk. (Accessed January 2010.)

Borys, D. S. & Pope, K. S. (1989) Dual relationships between therapist and client: a national study of psychologists, psychiatrists and social workers. *Professional Psychology: Research and Practice*, **20**, 283–293.

Bouhoutsos, J. (1985) Sexual intimacy between psychotherapists and clients: policy implications for the future. In *Women and Mental Health Policy* (ed. L. Walker), pp. 207–227. Sage.

Bouhoutsos, J., Holroyd, J. Lerman, H., *et al* (1983) Sexual intimacy between psychotherapists and patients. *Professional Psychology: Research and Practice*, **14**, 185–196.

Butler, S. & Zelen, S. L. (1977) Sexual intimacies between therapists and patients. *Psychotherapy: Theory, Research and Practice*, **14**, 139–145.

Coleman, P. (1988) Sex between psychiatrist and former patient: a proposal for a 'no harm, no foul' rule. *Oklahoma Law Review*, **41**, 1–52.

Department of Health (2005) *The Kerr/Haslam Inquiry*. The Stationery Office.

Derosis, H., Hamilton, J. A., Morrison, E., *et al* (1987) More on psychiatrist–patient sexual contact. *American Journal of Psychiatry*, **144**, 688–689.

Donaldson, L. (1994) Doctors with problems in an NHS workforce. *BMJ*, **308**, 1277–1182.

Edwards, D. J. A. (1981) The role of touch in interpersonal relations: implications for psychotherapy. *South African Journal of Psychology*, **11**, 29–37.

Garrett, T. & Davis, J. (1998) The prevalence of sexual contact between British clinical psychologists and their patients. *Clinical Psychology and Psychotherapy*, **5**, 253–263.

Gartrell, N., Herman, J., Olarte, S., *et al* (1986) Psychiatrist–patient sexual contact: results of a national survey, I: prevalence. *American Journal of Psychiatry*, **143**, 1126–1131.

Gartrell, N., Herman, J., Olarte, S., *et al* (1987) Reporting practices of psychiatrists who knew of sexual misconduct by colleagues. *American Journal of Orthopsychiatry*, **57**, 287–295.

Gechtman, L. (1989) Sexual contact between social workers and their clients. In *Sexual Exploitation in Professional Relationships* (ed. G. O. Gabbard), pp. 27–38. American Psychiatric Press.

Goodman, M. & Teicher, A. (1988) To touch or not to touch. *Psychotherapy*, **25**, 492–500.

Gottlieb, M. C., Sell, J. M. & Schoenfeld, L. S. (1988) Social/romantic relationships with present and former clients: state licensing board actions. *Professional Psychology: Research and Practice*, **19**, 459–462.

Grunebaum, H. (1986) Harmful psychotherapy experiences. *American Journal of Psychotherapy*, **40**, 165–176.

Holroyd, J. C. & Brodsky, A. M. (1977) Psychologists' attitudes and practices regarding erotic and nonerotic physical contact with patients. *American Psychologist*, **32**, 843–849.

Holroyd, J. C. & Brodsky, A. M. (1980) Does touching patients lead to sexual intercourse? *Professional Psychology*, **11**, 807–811.

Holub, E. A. & Lee, S. S. (1990) Therapists' use of nonerotic physical contact: ethical concerns. *Professional Psychology: Research and Practice*, **21**, 115–117.

Jehu, D. (1994) *Patients as Victims: Sexual Abuse in Psychotherapy and Counselling*. Wiley.

Kardener, S., Fuller, M. & Mensh, I. (1973) A survey of physicians' attitudes and practices regarding erotic and nonerotic contact with patients. *American Journal of Psychiatry*, **130**, 1077–1081.

Kardener, S., Fuller, M. & Mensh, I. (1976) Characteristics of 'erotic' practitioners. *American Journal of Psychiatry*, **133**, 1324–1325.

Kertay, L. & Reviere, S. L. (1993) The use of touch in psychotherapy: theoretical and ethical considerations. *Psychotherapy*, **30**, 32–48.

Kuchan, A. (1989) Survey of incidence of psychotherapists' sexual contact with clients in Wisconsin. In *Psychotherapists' Sexual Involvement with Clients: Intervention and Prevention* (eds G. R. Schoener, J. H. Milgrom, J. C. Gonsoriek, *et al*), pp. 51–64. Minneapolis Walk-In Counselling Center.

Mogul, K. M. (1992) Ethics complaints against female psychiatrists. *American Journal of Psychiatry*, **149**, 651–653.

Paufley, A. (2004) *Committee of Inquiry: Independent Investigation into How the NHS Handled Allegations About the Conduct of Clifford Ayling*. Department of Health.

Perr, I. N. (1989) Medicolegal aspects of professional sexual exploitation. In *Sexual Exploitation in Professional Relationships* (ed. G. O. Gabbard), pp. 211–228. American Psychiatric Press.

Perry, J. A. (1976) Physicians' erotic and nonerotic physical involvement with patients. *American Journal of Psychiatry*, **133**, 838–840.

Pope, K. S. (1993) Licensing disciplinary actions for psychologists who have been sexually involved with a client: some information about offenders. *Professional Psychology: Research and Practice*, **24**, 374–377.

Pope, K. S. & Bouhoutsos, J. C. (1986) *Sexual Intimacy between Therapists and Patients.* Praeger.

Pope, K. S. & Feldman-Summers, S. (1992) National survey of psychologists' sexual and physical abuse history and their evaluation of training and competence in these areas. *Professional Psychology: Research and Practice*, **23**, 353–361.

Pope, K. S. & Tabachnick, B. G. (1993) Therapists' anger, hate, fear, and sexual feelings: national survey of therapist responses, client characteristics, critical events, formal complaints, and training. *Professional Psychology: Research and Practice*, **24**, 142–152.

Pope, K. S. & Vetter, V. A. (1991) Prior therapist–patient sexual involvement among patients seen by psychologists. *Psychotherapy*, **28**, 429–438.

Pope, K. S., Levenson, H. & Schover, L. R. (1979) Sexual intimacy in psychology training: results and implications of a national survey. *American Psychologist*, **34**, 682–689.

Pope, K. S., Keith-Spiegel, P. & Tabachnick, B. G. (1986) Sexual attraction to clients: the human therapist and the (sometimes) inhuman training system. *American Psychologist*, **41**, 147–158.

Pope, K. S., Tabachnick, B. G. & Keith-Spiegel, P. (1987) Ethics of practice: the beliefs and behaviours of psychologists as therapists. *American Psychologist*, **42**, 993–1006.

Quadrio, C. (1996) Sexual abuse in therapy: gender issues. *Australian and New Zealand Journal of Psychiatry*, **30**, 124–133.

Rodolfa, E., Hall, T., Holms, V., *et al* (1994) The management of sexual feelings in therapy. *Professional Psychology: Research and Practice*, **25**, 168–172.

Russell, J. (1993) *Out of Bounds: Sexual Exploitation in Counselling and Therapy.* Sage.

Sarkar, S. P. (2004) Boundary violations and sexual exploitation in psychiatry and psychotherapy: a review. *Advances in Psychiatric Treatment*, **10**, 312–320.

Schoener, G. R. (1991) Therapist–client sexual involvement – incidence and prevalence. *Minnesota Psychologist*, January, 14–15.

Sonne, J. L. & Pope, K. S. (1991) Treating victims of therapist–patient sexual involvement. *Psychotherapy*, **28**, 174–187.

Sonne, J., Meyer, C. B., Borys, D., *et al* (1985) Clients' reactions to sexual intimacy in therapy. *American Journal of Orthopsychiatry*, **55**, 183–189.

Stake, J. E. & Oliver, J. (1991) Sexual contact and touching between therapist and client: a survey of psychologists' attitudes and behaviour. *Professional Psychology: Research and Practice*, **22**, 297–307.

Thoreson, R. W., Shaughnessy, P., Heppner, P. P., *et al* (1993) Sexual contact during and after the therapeutic relationship: attitudes and practices of male counsellors. *Journal of Counseling and Development*, **71**, 429–434.

Vinson, J. S. (1987) Use of complaint procedures in cases of therapist–patient sexual contact. *Professional Psychology: Research and Practice*, **18**, 159–164.

Williams, M. H. (1992) Exploitation and interference: mapping the damage from therapist–patient sexual involvement. *American Psychologist*, **47**, 412–421.

CHAPTER 6

Psychiatry: responding to the Kerr/Haslam Inquiry

Fiona Subotsky

Overview

The focus of the Kerr/Haslam Inquiry was on the handling of concerns raised about two consultant psychiatrists. This chapter looks at the information provided to the Inquiry by the Royal College of Psychiatrists and its subsequent response to the issues raised.

Introduction

The Kerr/Haslam Inquiry was set up by the Secretary of State for Health in 2002 under the chairmanship of Nigel Pleming QC. Its remit was to look at how the National Health Service (NHS) handled allegations regarding the performance and conduct of two consultant psychiatrists who worked for the same psychiatric hospital in York, north Yorkshire, in the 1970s and 1980s (Department of Health, 2005). In 2000 William Kerr had been convicted (in his absence, on a trial of the facts) of one count of indecent assault; by 2003 Michael Haslam had been convicted of four counts of indecent assault, and a conviction of rape had been quashed on appeal. Complaints had apparently been received over many years, with little to no response, and more complainants came forward during the course of the Inquiry. The details of the complaints are quoted from the Inquiry report in Boxes 6.1 and 6.2.

Request for information by the inquiry

The Royal College of Psychiatrists (RCPsych) was formally asked for comments on its policies and views over the period 1961–2004. What

Box 6.1 The complaints against Michael Haslam

Michael Haslam took up his post as Consultant in Psychological Medicine at Clifton Hospital, York, and Harrogate District Hospital in 1970. ...

During the course of the Inquiry we received evidence indicating that at least eight patients had, during his time in York, raised concerns about his alleged sexual advances towards them. Many of the allegations involved offering friendship and social activities outside of the clinical setting, leading later to the development of a personal, sexual relationship. ...

The number of patients who have subsequently come forward alleging that they were sexually propositioned or assaulted by Michael Haslam brings the total number of those who have now made allegations against him to at least 10.

The first complaint against Michael Haslam known to us occurred in 1974 when Patient B1 informed her GP, that (allegedly) she had been having an affair with Michael Haslam. However, in a pattern that echoed the response to complaints regarding William Kerr, this was never pursued either by the patient herself or by [the general practitioner] as a formal complaint or as an issue that needed to be reported to health service management – even with the identity of the patient concealed.

... concerns continued to be raised throughout his career. ...

Michael Haslam practised a range of treatments not widely known about or used within mental health settings. One such treatment was full-body massage (carried out without a chaperone). The Inquiry heard evidence on how on occasions this was carried out in isolated parts of the hospital or out of hours. ...

In three cases attempts were made to commence a formal complaint by means of letters ... or a written statement. However, in none of the cases did matters progress to an investigation, no patient apparently being prepared to go through with a formal complaints procedure.

Source: Department of Health (2005).

follows in this section is an abridged version of the response by the author on behalf of the College.

Background

In 1971 the RCPsych was set up, having evolved from the Royal Medico-Psychological Association. Its stated objects were:

1   to advance the science and practice of psychiatry and related subjects
2   to further public education therein
3   to promote study and research work in psychiatry and all sciences and disciplines connected with the understanding and treatment of mental disorder in all its forms and aspects and related subjects and publish the results of all such study and research.

Box 6.2 The complaints against William Kerr

The first complaint against William Kerr in North Yorkshire was in his very first year in [his consultant] post, 1965. This, as with so many subsequent cases, was communicated by a patient to her GP. However, in a pattern that was to be repeated many times, no formal complaint was lodged by the patient with the hospital authorities or with William Kerr's employer, nor did any GP take the initiative to pursue the matter. The complaint progressed no further than forming part of the reserve of knowledge of one particular GP. ...

However, this was not the first time an allegation of sexual misconduct had been raised. William Kerr had left his previous post in Northern Ireland in 1964 after an internal disciplinary hearing concerning an allegation of inappropriate sexual conduct with a patient (the details of which remain unclear). ...

Concerns continued to be raised about William Kerr throughout his career. The accounts we heard from patients were strikingly similar. The allegations were of unscheduled domiciliary visits, or appointments being arranged for the end of clinics when there would be few nursing staff around. William Kerr would then allegedly expose himself and 'invite' patients to perform sexual acts (often of masturbation or oral sex) upon him, sometimes suggesting that this was part of their treatment. A number of patients also alleged that full sexual intercourse took place. A number of women described William Kerr's ability to make them comply with his wishes, leaving them confused and guilty about their own actions and afraid to complain in forthright terms. ...

In the period prior to 1983, of the 30 concerns alleged to have been raised about William Kerr all but one fell on deaf ears.

Source: Department of Health (2005).

Thus, the focus of the College is primarily educational rather than regulatory.

RCPsych membership and disciplinary procedures

Membership was to be gained by examination after an approved training course; subsequently, active membership was maintained by annual subscription. Membership could be terminated if there were erasure from the Medical Register of the General Medical Council (GMC) or equivalent. If a member were suspended from such a register on grounds other than of ill-health, or had been convicted of a criminal offence, or 'acted in any respect in a dishonourable or unprofessional manner', or was otherwise unfit, the case could be brought to the RCPsych Court of Electors, which could recommend termination of membership, with the right of appeal to Council. Up to 2004, 19 members had had their membership of the College terminated, mainly following erasure from the GMC Register, but also following serious criminal conviction.

Awareness of boundary issues

The impropriety of doctor–patient sexual contact was traditionally taught in medical school and dates from Hippocrates (see Chapter 4). It was regarded as the province of the GMC to set the standard and to take action as necessary after notification. In relation to the specialty, the Mental Health Act 1959 specified that sexual intercourse with patients was an offence (section 128). At this time, the poor conduct of individual doctors could also be brought to the attention of the then 'Three Wise Men' system or to the regional medical officer. Nevertheless, the ethos of not complaining about the actions of other doctors was strong.

Awareness of institutional abuse was highlighted through various scandals, which led to inquiries and eventually the setting up of the Hospital Advisory Service in 1969. On the whole, the focus was on physical abuse and neglect, though doubtless sexual boundary breaking would also have occurred. During this period there was also increasing awareness of the sexual abuse of children, previously undisclosed or not believed. The 1970s and 1980s were also the period of both 'the sexual revolution', in which conventional ideas of sexual morality were questioned, and of feminist ideas, which began to question whether the comparative powerlessness of women within mental health systems led to a variety of misdiagnoses and mistreatments.

In the psychiatric curriculum, formal psychodynamic psychotherapy training would have been the most likely place to bring up issues of emotions between patient and doctor using the concepts of transference and countertransference. There was not, however, a requirement for such training.

College policies and publications

In the late 1980s and early 1990s, there were five publications or College documents of relevance:

1   The registrar's 'Statement on abuse and harassment within psychiatric hospitals' (Gath, 1989) noted that 'incidents involving sexual harassment of patients in psychiatric hospitals have been brought to the notice of the Public Policy Committee'. Brief recommendations were made regarding security, education of patients and training of staff; there was no specific allusion to abuse of patients by staff.
2   Subotsky (1991), in a paper entitled 'Issues for women in the development of mental health services', noted two important relevant emergent themes: the lessons from child sexual abuse about listening to – and believing – the victim; and the importance of the role of the consumer, as patient or carer, in influencing the health services received.
3   In a later paper, 'Sexual abuse in psychiatric hospitals: developing policies to aid prevention', Subotsky (1993) presented simplified policies on this topic and a specific reference was made to the action

to be taken in the event of an allegation that a member of staff had committed a sexual assault – specifically, reporting and ensuring disciplinary procedures were followed.

4   This was taken further by a College Council Report of 1996, *Sexual Abuse and Harassment in Psychiatric Settings*. That report stated: 'It has been suggested that abuse/harassment perpetrated by psychiatric staff involves 5–9% of staff … [there is] continual pressure on the staff to get caught up in psychopathology. … People may seek out employment where the vulnerable may be exploited … there needs to be an effective policy of vetting staff and volunteers'.

5   In the 1998 publication *Seminars in Psychosexual Disorders*, West (1998), a chapter entitled 'Problems of sexuality among people in mental health facilities' elaborated on the issue of sexual contact between staff and patients as follows:

[It] should be explicitly prohibited and defined as a serious disciplinary offence. This necessarily goes beyond what is forbidden by criminal law, which penalises intercourse with a patient only if the perpetrator is male and the patient female and is silent on the issue of consensual acts other than intercourse. Complaints … are quite common. … All institutions need a written policy with procedures clearly laid down. … A distressed victim has a right to have the incident properly established.

Subsequently, the GMC brought to the College's attention the fact that allegations about sexual impropriety were being made against psychiatrists, and it asked for the development of specific standards. This was to facilitate judgement about what was appropriate and inappropriate, specifically in this area but also with respect to amplification of the GMC's document *Good Medical Practice* (General Medical Council, 2001). In response, the College developed the following two policy documents, which were circulated to all members:

1   *Good Psychiatric Practice* (Royal College of Psychiatrists, 2000). Of particular relevance here was the section on the 'trusting relationship' (pp. 7–9): 'The psychiatrist will … respect patients' privacy and dignity … be mindful of the vulnerability of some patients to exploitation within the therapeutic relationship'; and within the psychotherapy section, 'Good practice in psychotherapy will include … paying particular attention to boundaries, time and place, and being sensitive to the psychological implications of transgressing boundaries, e.g. through touch or self-revelation'.

2   *Vulnerable Patients, Vulnerable Doctors. Good Practice in Our Clinical Relationships* (Royal College of Psychiatrists, 2002). This document included three key points in its summary:

•   Physical contact may be perceived as an appropriate comfort in some situations and as an assault in others. What matters is the meaning of the doctor's behaviour for the patient, not the innocence of the doctor's intentions.

- Relationships of sexual intimacy between doctor and patient are totally unacceptable. Both patient and doctor will be protected by the use of chaperones where misinterpretation is possible.
- Innovative techniques should be used only if there is good evidence as to their propriety and effectiveness, with the consent of the patient and with full preparation.

Complaints

Initially there was no formal system within the College to deal with complaints from either patients or other professionals. General issues brought to the attention of staff or officers would have been redirected to the employer, the service or the GMC, while the Mental Health Act Commission, established in 1983, had a specific remit to look at the complaints of detained patients.

In 1999 an information phone-line, open to the public as well as members, was established in the College library service. Some patient complaints were made directly to the College via this route; these were generally redirected to the appropriate authority, such as the NHS trust involved or the GMC. By 2004 disciplinary and complaints procedures had been reviewed, especially in relation to what was appropriate for the College to regulate rather than the GMC. It was agreed to concentrate on issues to do with College roles and functions. Thus the removal of appointments as Tutor, Examiner, or of Honorary Officer would be possible.

Psychosexual therapies

The archives held very little reference to psychosexual therapies apart from the publication *Seminars in Psychosexual Disorders* (Freeman *et al*, 1998). Clinics were often held in conjunction with other services, such as urology, family planning or gynaecology. Training courses were not provided by the College, although some consideration had been given to this in 1981, in conjunction with the Royal College of Obstetricians and Gynaecologists. Some knowledge of psychosexual problems and treatment was expected in the membership examination. The issue of chaperonage was not especially emphasised. Anecdotally, in the 1970s and 1980s, with general lessening of formality on the one hand and resource pressures on the other, the possibility and awareness of advisability of chaperone use for intimate and other physical examinations decreased across medical practice, including psychiatry. Nevertheless, physical examination, which could include intimate examination, was still considered to be an important part of general psychiatric initial and emergency assessment. During the 1970s the British Association for Sexual and Relationship Therapy was established, which involved psychiatrists, although there was no formal relationship with the College. It developed its own code of ethics (see Chapter 9).

Trust and NHS policies

During the 1990s much progress across the NHS was made in consulting the users of services (or 'consumers' or 'patients') and developing patient advocacy services. Formal complaints procedures, with appeal to the NHS ombudsman, became better known. Trusts had their own medical disciplinary policies and clear responsibility through clinical governance for the quality of the service they provided. Viewing allegations of boundary breaches as a 'risk issue' (for instance because of the possibility of litigation) had also helped bring the issue into focus. Mental health services for women had been separately considered by the NHS, and there was greater emphasis on providing safety for in-patients.

General observations

Within psychiatric services, unjustified allegations are not uncommon, but it must not be assumed that all allegations are so, especially if there is a pattern to them. Many adult patients are likely to have a history of sexual abuse, and while this might make false allegations more likely, it could also increase the patient's vulnerability to actual further abuse.

Preventing sexual abuse of psychiatric patients is highly relevant for training and service provision. Risk factors in institutions are better known than they were: isolation, non-capacitous or non-verbal patients, poor layout and staffing, hostility to 'whistle-blowing', poor attention to complaints from patients on grounds of their disturbance, bullying and denying staff attitudes. However, it is clear that the closure of large institutions did not always end such problems, as they could also occur in small institutions and indeed out-patient services. Policies for staff need to be explicit.

Governance policies, including appraisal of consultants, the requirement for continuous professional development, and an emphasis on audit and evidence-based treatments, should help to promote good practice. However, psychiatry is a specialty of high need but great shortage, which may affect managerial capacity to deal with difficult issues. The use of locums and the regulation of private practice present particular difficulties in maintaining quality. Within the NHS the right to a second opinion is a valuable one and should be respected, even if there is a shortage of resources and apparent catchment-area problems.

Process of the Kerr/Haslam Inquiry and subsequent College action

The Inquiry heard evidence from those involved, commissioned specialist reports, and held two seminars at which the key themes identified were discussed with a wide range of stakeholders. The author attended as the formal representative of the College, while other members of the College provided specialist reports and contributed to the debates as individual experts. Meetings took place largely in 2004; the final report was presented in 2005.

Review of GMC cases involving psychiatrists

Following this, and in order for the RCPsych to have a better understanding of the situation *vis-à-vis* psychiatrists, the author reviewed the GMC website for reports of psychiatrists about whom the Professional Conduct Committee (PCC) concluded its deliberations in the period January 2000 to November 2004, when the procedure was altered. Table 6.1 gives a brief description of the sexual misconduct issues and the hearing outcomes. There were 19 cases of sexual misconduct considered sufficiently serious and well founded to take to the PCC, all involving men. In comparison there were 17 PCC hearings concerning other issues, of which the most common was improper prescribing; two of these cases involved women. Two doctors had offended in a different country and moved to the UK.

It is evident that, over this period, sexual misconduct was the major issue for serious professional misconduct (SPM) hearings at the GMC for psychiatrists. While it is not possible to compare the data with those for other specialties, it is clear that a range of behaviour is covered, with a range of outcomes.

RCPsych response to the recommendations

Issues on which the College might take action were suggested both in the discussions at the stakeholders' meetings and in the final recommendations of the Inquiry.

A code of ethics

The Inquiry chairman was concerned that the College should consider developing a code of ethics (as suggested by Sarkar & Adshead, 2003), partly to clarify what could be appropriately considered grounds for disciplinary action, and to define whether sexual relationships with 'former patients' should be permissible and if so under what circumstances. The College view, largely accepted by the chairman, was that the documents mentioned above corresponded to the GMC's *Good Medical Practice*, with further elaboration on the issue of vulnerability, but that they should be reviewed and revised.

On the issue of the lifelong ban on forming sexual relationships with former patients, other psychiatric associations have made this ruling because of the special nature of the psychotherapeutic relationship (see Appendix 2), even where the corresponding medical regulatory body has not required this of all doctors. It was agreed that the College's Clinical Governance Committee would include the former Ethics Committee in its remit and would specifically issue recommendations on this issue (see below).

Table 6.1 GMC Professional Conduct Committee: serious professional misconduct (SPM) hearings involving psychiatrists, 2000–04

Type of misconduct	Outcome of hearing
Sexual misconduct with patients	
Conviction of rape and assaults on patients	Erasure
Sex with patient	Erasure
Impropriety, 2 patients	Erasure
Impropriety, 1 patient	Erasure
Sexual assaults on male patients; conviction	Erasure
Impropriety with 1 patient in Australia. Concealed Australian findings	Erasure
Sexual relationship with 1 patient and approaching 2 others	Erasure
Impropriety, 1 patient	Erasure
Sexual relationship with patient despite warning	Erasure
Impropriety, 2 patients in Australia	Erasure
Impropriety, 3 patients	Erasure
Impropriety and inappropriate prescribing	Suspension
Impropriety and dishonesty	Conditions
Manner inappropriate and improper with 2 patients	SPM not found
Sexual relationship with patient	SPM not found
Other sexual misconduct	
Conviction of sexual offences with children	Erasure
Web child pornography; misrepresentation	Erasure
Inappropriate behaviour to female staff; inadequate patient examination	Suspension
Child pornography possession conviction	Suspension
Prescribing	
Prescribing	Erasure
Prescribing	Erasure
Prescribing	Erasure
Prescribing	Conditions
Prescribing	Conditions
Prescribing	Conditions
Prescribing	Conditions
Other	
Dishonesty	Erasure
Conviction for insurance fraud	Erasure
Misrepresentation	Erasure
Inadequate medication monitoring and inappropriate letters	Suspension
Fraud	Suspension
Conviction for driving offence	Conditions
Breaching confidentiality	Reprimand
Inappropriate reports and failure to discuss concerns	Reprimand
Child protection allegations about another doctor	SPM not found
Breach of confidentiality	SPM not found

Research into prevalence

The College had reservations about the potential usefulness of self-report member surveys of sexualised behaviour between doctors and existing or former patients (see Chapter 5 for a discussion of prevalence evidence), especially since such relationships had been made potentially criminal under the Sexual Offences Act 2003, but recommended the better collection and analysis of data from third-party reporting systems such as NHS trust complaints and incidents and referrals to the GMC.

Centralised records

The Inquiry recommended some form of central recording linked to the named professional, which would include non-proven allegations. Although this approach had had some success in sexual offence prosecutions, the likelihood of false allegations and the suggestion of easy access to such data make this approach problematic. Even though the GMC could adopt such a system, it would not include the many mental health workers who are not professionally registered, although the system of checking with the Criminal Records Bureau could usefully be extended.

Physical examinations and the use of chaperones

The Clinical Governance Committee offered further advice on the use of chaperones in the revised edition of *Vulnerable Patients, Vulnerable Doctors* (Royal College of Psychiatrists, 2002).

Treatments

The Inquiry warned against the use of 'unorthodox' treatments without good explanation, consent and monitoring, an issue again picked up in *Vulnerable Patients, Vulnerable Doctors* (Royal College of Psychiatrists, 2002).

Recruitment practices

Previous formal inquiries suggested that a number of sexual abuse incidents could be prevented if good recruitment practices were followed, including the vetting of agency and non-clinical staff. The Kerr/Haslam Inquiry recommended that one of the referees in any job application should be the consultant who conducts the applicant's appraisal, the clinical director or the medical director, and that references should be obtained from the three most recent employers and should be 'properly checked'. It was recommended that this should be part of the training and advice given to College assessors on consultant advisory appointment committees.

Staff performance

The RCPsych was in agreement with the recommendation for a '360 degree' appraisal system. A College-supported system was introduced in 2005 and it was suggested that clinical supervision systems for senior clinicians could be introduced through the peer-group system used in continuing professional development, although other models would be possible.

Training

The Inquiry recommended that all health workers should be able to discuss feelings of sexual attraction without the automatic risk of disciplinary action and that boundary issues should be part of the curriculum. The College Psychotherapy Faculty proposed developing further ideas and the topic was included at subsequent annual meetings. A useful educational review on the issue of professionals' abuse of patients was provided by Sarkar (2004).

RCPsych policy

The Inquiry had hoped that the College might act as a separate regulatory body, with compulsory membership, and complaints and sanction systems. While compulsion was not under the College's control, its view was that membership or affiliation to the College should be broadened as widely as possible and NHS trusts encouraged to employ staff with professional membership. Because there were already many other pathways for taking action against poorly performing doctors, which could lead to confusion, the disciplinary and complaints procedures were revised to focus on College-related activities. Meetings were held with the GMC and the National Clinical Advisory Service (NCAS) to clarify respective roles and expectations if complaints were received, whether from patients or professionals.

Patient information and support

The College supported the Inquiry's recommendations that NHS trusts should provide patients with information on what to expect in psychiatric assessment and treatment, how to make complaints, and how to access sources of independent advocacy and support. Within the College, increasing use was made of user and carer involvement in committees, projects and training. Queries from patients are received by the Library and Information Service, which is able to respond directly or to redirect people to more appropriate organisations, although it is not a clinical 'help-line' as such.

Subsequent developments

Policy

The College currently has a Clinical Governance Committee, with an Ethics Subcommittee, and a Policy Committee to consider new policy proposals. The *Vulnerable Patients* document was revised again as *Vulnerable Patients, Safe Doctors: Good Practice in Our Clinical Relationships* (CR 146; Royal College of Psychiatrists, 2007a). Principles of good practice in the variety of therapeutic relationships are discussed, and fictional vignettes are provided for consideration. Its Appendix, 'Avoiding boundary violations in psychiatric practice' includes a clear statement that 'Sexual relationships with patients or former patients are unethical and unacceptable' (reproduced here as Appendix 1). The third edition of *Good Psychiatric Practice* was published in 2009 (Royal College of Psychiatrists, 2009).

The original College report *Sexual Abuse and Harassment in Psychiatric Settings* (Royal College of Psychiatrists, 1996) was reviewed at length, and amended to take into account major developments in the legal framework within which patients are treated and to encompass a broader discussion of sexuality, with a recognition that clinicians have to balance principles of autonomy and protection. The possibility of staff abuse of patients must be recognised, and a number of recommendations are made which should help prevent this. The revised version, *Sexual Boundary Issues in Psychiatric Settings* (CR145; Royal College of Psychiatrists, 2007*b*), is available on the College website.

Disciplinary and complaints procedures

Currently, the Education, Training and Standards Committee, which has replaced the old Court of Electors, is responsible for the procedures governing termination of membership and other disciplinary action such as suspension or censure, following the regulations laid down in the College's bye-laws (Royal College of Psychiatrists, 2008). A complaints procedure is being developed.

Education

Boundary violation has been a recurrent topic of educational presentations at the annual meetings, and the College has an online series of educational modules (CPD Online) available to members. These include:

- Professional ethics and sexual boundary violations
- Appraisal for psychiatrists
- The physical examination in psychiatric practice
- Private practice for psychiatrists – practical, financial, legal and ethical issues
- An ethical framework for psychiatry
- Problem psychiatrists and what should be covered in suspension.

Whistle-blowing

There are evident difficulties for professionals who are potential 'proxy complainants' or whistle-blowers. The GMC's advice on this has been considerably amplified, but difficulties in reporting suspicions about a senior figure remain, especially if the patient has not given consent. The College would be supportive of any member in this situation through its Psychiatrists' Support Service, which provides confidential telephone advice, and has published a leaflet *On Whistle-Blowing and Passing On Concerns,* also available online (Psychiatrists' Support Service, 2008).

Conclusion

The topic of sexual and other abuse of patients by doctors had attracted little attention in the UK until the 1990s, though research elsewhere (see Chapter 5) had indicated it was not unusual and that psychiatrists were one of the groups most likely to be involved. The process of the Kerr/Haslam Inquiry usefully highlighted this as a comparatively unaddressed issue, with the GMC and RCPsych both being closely involved. All the recommendations of the Inquiry were seriously considered by the College, which subsequently clarified its policies, revised its decision-making processes, developed education and support methods, and improved liaison with other responsible agencies. However, there should not be complacency; specific teaching about how to handle the risks of patient–doctor encounters should be incorporated into the medical student curriculum, and enhanced in specialty training. Monitoring by the College and GMC of disciplinary cases would also be advantageous.

Acknowledgement

This chapter is an extended version of 'Responding to the Kerr/Haslam Inquiry' (Subotsky, 2006).

References

Department of Health (2005) *The Kerr/Haslam Inquiry.* London: TSO (The Stationery Office).

Freeman, H., Pullen, I. & Stein, G. (eds) (1998) *Seminars in Psychosexual Disorders.* Gaskell.

Gath, A. (1989) Statement on abuse and harassment within psychiatric hospitals. *Psychiatric Bulletin,* **13**, 460.

General Medical Council (2001) *Good Medical Practice.* GMC.

General Medical Council (2006) *Good Medical Practice* (4th edn). GMC. Online at http://www.gmc-uk.org/guidance/good_medical_practice/index.asp (accessed June 2010).

Psychiatrists' Support Service (2008) *On Whistle-Blowing and Passing On Concerns.* Pamphlet. Royal College of Psychiatrists.

Royal College of Psychiatrists (1996) *Sexual Abuse and Harassment in Psychiatric Settings* (Council Report CR52). Royal College of Psychiatrists.

Royal College of Psychiatrists (2000) *Good Psychiatric Practice* (Council Report CR83). Royal College of Psychiatrists.

Royal College of Psychiatrists (2001) *Supplemental Charter, By-Laws and Regulations* (Occasional Paper OP52). Royal College of Psychiatrists.

Royal College of Psychiatrists (2002) *Vulnerable Patients, Vulnerable Doctors. Good Practice in Our Clinical Relationships* (Council Report CR101). Royal College of Psychiatrists.

Royal College of Psychiatrists (2007*a*) *Vulnerable Patients, Safe Doctors: Good Practice in Our Clinical Relationships* (Council Report CR146). Royal College of Psychiatrists.

Royal College of Psychiatrists (2007*b*) *Sexual Boundary Issues in Psychiatric Settings* (Council Report CR145). Royal College of Psychiatrists.

Royal College of Psychiatrists (2008) *Supplemental Charter, Bye-Laws and Regulations* (Occasional Paper OP68). Royal College of Psychiatrists.

Royal College of Psychiatrists (2009) *Good Psychiatric Practice* (3rd edn) (Council Report CR154). Royal College of Psychiatrists.

Sarkar, S. P. (2004) Boundary violation and sexual exploitation in psychiatry and psychotherapy: a review. *Advances in Psychiatric Treatment*, **10**, 312–320.

Sarkar, S. P. & Adshead, G. (2003) Protecting altruism: a call for a code of ethics in British psychiatry. *British Journal of Psychiatry*, **183**, 95–97.

Subotsky, F. (1991) Issues for women in the development of mental health services. *British Journal of Psychiatry*, **158** (suppl. 10), 17–21.

Subotsky, F. (1993) Sexual abuse in psychiatric hospitals: developing policies to aid prevention. *Psychiatric Bulletin*, **17**, 274–276.

Subotsky, F. (2006) Responding to the Kerr/Haslam Inquiry. *Psychiatric Bulletin*, **30**, 207–209.

West, D. J. (1998) Problems of sexuality among people in mental health facilities. In *Seminars in Psychosexual Disorders* (eds H. Freeman, I. Pullen, G. Stein, *et al*), pp. 124–141. Gaskell.

CHAPTER 7

The general practitioner and abuse in primary care

David Misselbrook

Overview

UK general practice has its own particular culture. While using a holistic medical model, general practitioners (GPs) also have to be business minded and act as gatekeepers to secondary care services. This creates some inevitable tensions between GPs' and patients' interests. A particular problem is treading the line between benign and potentially abusive paternalism. General practice has provided an environment in which spectacular abuses may rarely occur. This chapter looks first at the environment of the doctor–patient interaction and its relevance to patient abuse and then at specific instances of patient abuse in general practice.

Constructing the environment of the doctor–patient interaction in general practice

General practice culture

The gulf between the practice of medicine in hospitals and in the community is particularly deep in the UK. This gulf was institutionalised by the creation of the National Health Service (NHS) in 1948: hospital doctors became state employees but general practitioners (GPs) retained their independent contractor status and this had a profound and enduring effect on the culture of general practice.

General practitioners practise medicine in the community while at the same time running a small business. This will be a familiar tension to groups of private specialists, but not to most hospital consultants or juniors. Thus GPs typically work in partnerships that employ other staff, such as nurses, receptionists, clerical staff and practice managers. The local primary care trust (PCT) pays gross sums to the partnership as determined by the size of the practice, whether various targets are reached and what additional services are provided. The partnership must then pay their staff, provide premises if they choose to practise from their own building, and pay all other costs. The profits then remaining are divided between the partners as they themselves have determined in the partnership agreement.

General practice is carried out at a cottage industry scale, rather than the typical industrial scale of activity of the average hospital. GPs tend to be professionally embedded in their communities, and practise a form of medicine that consciously embraces a biopsychosocial model, both of pathology and of care. They may know their patients and their patients' families as their lives unfold together over decades. GPs form one part of the wider primary healthcare team, which also includes healthcare workers employed directly by PCTs and other bodies, for example health visitors, community nurses, community occupational therapists and family planning clinic doctors.

General practitioners therefore tend to be both holistic and individualistic, and have a practical concern both for patients and for business. They consider their independence to be in their own and their patients' best interests. When UK general practice works well, it is rightly valued as a world-class model for primary care medicine. But, as with any large group of small individualistic bodies, there is also plenty of scope for things to go wrong and perhaps also remain hidden.

The elusive goal of patient-centred medicine

General practice culture puts a high value on patient-centred medicine. This is perhaps most clearly expressed by Tuckett *et al* (1985) in the classic book *Meetings Between Experts*. Tuckett's model recognises that the doctor is an expert in medicine, and that the patient is an expert on his or her own life, preferences, priorities and goals. The purpose of the consultation therefore becomes a dialectical process between these two separate areas of expertise, with the doctor ultimately seeking to use his or her medical knowledge to serve the patient's specific preferences and goals.

The problem with this best conceivable goal for medicine is that it is rarely fully achievable. The normal consultation lasts 10 minutes, during which time the GP must listen to the patient's problem, examine the patient as needed, explain and discuss any relevant medical factors, negotiate and agree a management plan, create a safety net strategy for when things do not go to plan, and deal with issues on the doctor's agenda such as health promotion. Thus patient-centred consultations often constitute 'front-of-house' models that we aspire to and teach our trainees, while 'back-stage' behaviour may be based more on compromise between such aspirations and the exigencies and pressures of the working environment (Fig. 7.1).

Hopefully, commitments to behave ethically and practise in a patient-centred way will markedly moderate self-interest. Shaw (1911) claimed that 'all professions are conspiracies against the laity'. How much is the

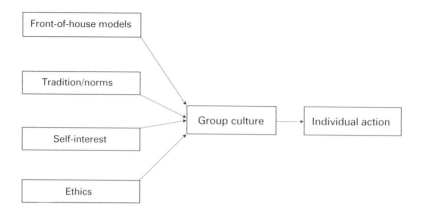

Fig. 7.1 The four main influences that determine general practitioners' behaviour.

profession of medicine structured for the benefit of patients, and how much is it structured for doctors' benefit? Wilmshurst (2000) asserts that 'clinical performance and welfare of patients often come second to the interests of institutions and loyalty to colleagues'. Freidson (1985) argues that doctors maintain professional dominance over patients by controlling an exclusive licence to practise medicine, prescribe drugs, refer to specialists and admit patients to hospital. Other doctors and clinical departments, by contrast, are seen as colleagues and collaborators.

Doctors hold a powerful monopoly (Berlant, 1975) and beyond the specific rights held exclusively by doctors is the broader cultural authority of medicine (Starr, 1982). Doctors normally hold the balance of power in the consulting rooms. Their ethics call on them to use that power for the good of patients, but they can hardly maintain that they never use any of it for their own comfort too – doctors make a comfortable living out of medicine. GPs are pushed by incentives, such as Quality and Outcome Framework (QOF) points, to skew their practice towards ways which the Department of Health (DH) has determined represent patients' interests. This leaves open the possibility of 'gaming' – practising in a way that is directed to getting the best figures rather than the best outcome for the individual patient. Therefore the challenge to doctors is to be open about how they practise and, as the General Medical Council (2004) requires, to strive always to 'make the care of your patient your first concern'. Doctors need to be committed to the care of individual patients as well as the care of populations. So if a computer prompts a check on the patient's smoking status and a reminder that her smear is overdue, one might need moral courage to mention neither issue if she is distressed and needing to talk about her son's drug habit.

This raises very practical questions as to whether GPs get the balance right between their own interest (e.g. the need to earn a reasonable living and have time for their families) and patients' interests. For example, it would be possible to run one's practice in a way that sought to maximise income yet minimise patient service. One of the criticisms of the pre-2003 GP contract was that it contained incentives which encouraged exactly this. In the new 2003 GP contract gaming is still possible. At what point does business-efficient practice become sharp practice, or poor practice become patient abuse?

Structural challenges

Some thinkers see the medical world as inherently (albeit unintentionally) abusive and re-analyse healthcare in terms of power relationships (Jewson, 1976). Such a discourse sees doctors as systematically disempowering patients and thus views medicine as constructing itself as a malign form of paternalism. It is worth briefly reflecting on such accounts as part of the context in which we should understand the concept of patient abuse.

Foucault

Michel Foucault (1926–84) conceived of history (and social activities such as sexuality, crime and punishment, and medicine) as a series of changing thought systems that determine our construction of the world and how we act within it. He was particularly concerned with the exercise of power within social systems, and explored the ways in which social control and discipline are constructed and maintained. He developed this theme through his definitive historical studies of human sexuality, of crime and punishment and of medicine. I do not present Foucault's views as 'facts' but as one side of an argument containing a kernel of truth we would do well to consider.

Foucault's *The Birth of the Clinic* (first published in 1963) should be read by all reflective doctors. Foucault develops the concept of 'the medical gaze', describing how doctors modify the patient's story, fitting it into a biomedical paradigm and filtering out non-biomedical material. Doctors systematically look at some bits of the story and exclude others. A 'gaze' is an act of selecting the elements of the total data stream available to our senses, and the way in which we perceive them (the *seeing-as* factor). It is attention plus interpretation. Foucault describes the medical gaze as 'no longer the gaze of any observer, but that of a doctor endowed with the power of decision and intervention' (Foucault, 1989, p. 89).

Foucault's charge is that doctors are doctor oriented, not patient oriented, and thus function within an abusive power structure. They tend to select out the biomedical bits of the patients' problems and ignore the rest. Medical school teaches them more about biomedicine than about patients. Moreover, the 'medical tribe' tends to dominate rather than negotiate. They control, stick people on trolleys, strand them in waiting rooms, put them in bed in silly gowns and talk above their heads.

Illich

Ivan Illich starts his major critique, *Medical Nemesis* (1976), with the assertion that 'the medical establishment has become a major threat to health'. He makes three claims:

1   Doctors are useless – their attempt to reduce society's burden of illness does not work. Along with many others I have refuted this elsewhere (Misselbrook, 2001).
2   Doctors have organised medicine for their own good, contrary to the interests of patients;
3   Doctors exert inappropriate social control by turning normal human problems into medical problems ('medical imperialism').

Thus, for both Foucault and Illich, the medical system is oppressive and tends to abuse patients' best interests.

Kennedy

A more specific challenge came from Ian Kennedy, who first voiced his deep scepticism of the UK system of medicine in his 1980 Reith lectures, 'Unmasking medicine' (published in book form by Kennedy, 1981). Kennedy is more recently known for his chairmanship of the Bristol Royal Infirmary Inquiry (relating to tertiary care). While Foucault and Illich painted a general background of sociological unease, Kennedy brought medicine's faults into the public spotlight.

The opening of the synopsis of the Bristol Inquiry report gives the flavour of Kennedy's charge against UK NHS medicine:

The story of the paediatric cardiac surgical service in Bristol is not an account of bad people. Nor is it an account of people who did not care, nor of people who wilfully harmed patients. It is an account of people who cared greatly about human suffering, and were dedicated and well-motivated. Sadly, some lacked insight and their behaviour was flawed. Many failed to communicate with each other, and to work together effectively for the interests of their patients. (Bristol Royal Infirmary Inquiry, 2001, p. 2)

Kennedy's synopsis continues with prophetic words:

For the future, it must be part of all healthcare professionals' contracts with a trust (and part of a GP's terms of service) that they undergo appraisal, continuing professional development and revalidation to ensure that all healthcare professionals remain competent to do their job. ... Doctors, nurses and managers must work together ... with clear lines of accountability, in order to provide the best possible care for patients ... there must be agreed and published standards of clinical care for healthcare professionals to follow, so that patients and the public know what to expect. (p. 3)

Thus, the general sociological critique followed by the specific cases of Bristol Royal Infirmary and Harold Shipman (see Box 7.1) sets the stage for the development of distrust of doctors in general and GPs in particular.

The role of burnout and sickness in patient abuse

In the UK Caplan (1994) found that 27% of GPs scored as depressed or borderline depressed on the Hospital Anxiety and Depression Scale (HAD scale) and 14% had suicidal thoughts. A report form the British Medical Medical Association (2000) found that 48% of GPs had suffered psychological distress, 14% had felt suicidal and 23% had used alcohol as a response to anxiety.

Does it matter if doctors are chronically stressed? Freudenberger (1974) coined the term 'burnout' to describe chronic work-related distress. Burnout is usually seen as having three separate but related components:

- emotional exhaustion
- depersonalisation of others
- reduced personal accomplishment.

Schattner (1998) found that when GPs were stressed, patient care suffered. Firth-Cozens & Greenhalgh (1997) found that over a third of both hospital doctors and GPs reported specific instances when patient care had been compromised through tiredness, overwork and depression. The actual effect depends very much upon the personal attributes of the individual doctor. McManus *et al* (2004) found that stress levels and burnout are determined by the doctors' personality and learning styles, and that these characteristics persist predictably over a decade of follow-up.

The intimate examination

Lief & Fox (1963) observed that the doctor has privileged access to a patient's body. Emerson (1970) stated that 'the physician is permitted to handle the patient's body in ways otherwise permitted only to special intimates, and in the case of procedures such as rectal and vaginal examinations in ways not even permitted to a sexual partner'. During a vaginal examination (VE), the doctor inserts his or her fingers into the woman's vagina, an area of the body that normally has a sexual context. This examination is therefore 'precarious' in its status as a non-emotive technical procedure. A VE is an example of the clash between the different worlds doctors and patients construct. Emerson comments that 'the gynaecological examination merely exaggerates the internally contradictory nature of definitions of reality found in most situations'.

To remain safe, the examination must be 'constructed' as a medical procedure, removed from the common connotations of such contact. The examination will usually be conducted in a 'medical space'. The doctor's behaviour and speech become stylised, as if the doctor as a person is not really there. Eye contact during the examination is often avoided, as if the patient as a person is not there either. Joking is unlikely, and superfluous or lingering contact avoided.

In cases such as Ayling (see Box 10.1, p. 115) and Green (see Box 7.2, below), the contextual fragility of such intimate examinations may form a specific point of vulnerability to patient abuse. Both doctor and patient run the risk of slipping towards experiencing such examinations within a sexual rather than clinical context. All doctors require a moral compass and a basic self-discipline not to cross this line within their own minds.

Specific problems of patient abuse in general practice

Researching abuse of patients by GPs is a depressing task: the reports produced by the General Medical Council (GMC) detail case after case of the moral failings of doctors in so many different ways. The case of Harold Shipman, discussed below, is an example of the extreme abuse of the power referred to by Foucault and was so grave that a public inquiry inevitably ensued. More commonplace scandals and failures of GPs are illustrated by the subsequent brief notes on some recent relevant GMC judgements.

Shipman

Harold Shipman was a mass murderer and, regrettably, an NHS GP. Drawing lessons from Shipman is not straightforward, as there can be no more extreme example of patient abuse. His behaviour lies so far outside any norm, even within the context of this book, that outrage kicks in, tending to obliterate reflective thought. Two remarkable features of his crimes are obvious, but bear consideration: that he killed so many and got away with it for so long. The case is outlined in Box 7.1.

The facts are presented in Dame Janet Smith's five-volume report (Smith, 2002). Although the Shipman case is extreme, there are some general lessons. A glaring warning sign occurred early on. In 1976 he was an opiate addict, misappropriating controlled drugs and was prosecuted for misuse of pethidine. However, he was not struck off the Medical Register. Shipman practised in partnership in the Donneybrook medical centre in Hyde from 1977 to 1992. He then left to move into single-handed practice in Market Street, Hyde. There were no obvious reasons for him to leave, and in retrospect one must assume that his criminal activities were relevant. Certainly he displayed some caution; there were episodes when he was concerned he might be under suspicion and he would then refrain from murder for some months. Overall, however, his rate of killing inexorably increased.

Box 7.1 Harold Shipman – mass murderer

Harold Shipman killed at least 215 patients between 1975 and 1998. The age range of his victims was 41–93 years. Of his confirmed victims, 171 were women and 44 were men. During this time he was a married family man. His wife had no idea that he was killing his patients. Shipman's typical *modus operandi* was to identify vulnerable elderly patients and inject them with intravenous diamorphine, either on home visits or occasionally in the surgery. He often falsified their records, for instance making it appear that they had recently been complaining of chest pains. He also apparently ended prematurely the lives of those with terminal disease. Some of those he killed he simply found inconvenient. He sometimes claimed to have found the patient dead and at other times would leave the scene for others to find the patient. He generally completed death certificates and cremation papers, stating that the patient had suffered an acute event such as a heart attack. Towards the end of his deadly career another local GP became suspicious at the number of Shipman's patients who died suddenly with Shipman around, and reported her suspicions. This led to a police investigation, which found no cause for concern – he had at this point killed about 200 patients.

Source: Smith (2002).

Shipman was hugely popular with his patients at both practices: 'he was held in very high regard by the overwhelming majority of his patients. He was also respected by fellow professionals. His patients appear to have regarded him as the best doctor in Hyde' (Smith, 2002, vol. 1, p. 181). He appeared authoritative and attentive, often visiting elderly patients even without a request. However, the Inquiry also found that Shipman displayed 'aggression, conceit, arrogance and contempt for those whom he considered to be his intellectual inferiors' (vol. 1, p. 184). He was also described as cold. Although he appears to have been thought well of by colleagues, he had no friends and did not socialise.

Shipman committed suicide in prison still denying his crimes, despite overwhelming evidence of his guilt, so we are left to speculate why he killed. Dame Janet Smith's view was that 'a person who has one addiction is quite likely to be subject to other forms of addiction. … It is possible that he was addicted to killing' (vol. 1, p. 187). Psychiatrists advising her 'made some tentative suggestions about his underlying personality but stress that these are only theories':

Shipman may have a rigid and obsessive personality … he may be isolated and may have difficulty in expressing emotions … his arrogance and over-confidence are almost certainly a mask for poor self-esteem … he was probably angry, deeply unhappy and chronically depressed. They suggest that he has a deep seated need to control people and events. Once he fears that he cannot control events, he feels threatened and reacts so as to take or regain control. (Smith, 2002, vol. 1, pp. 187–188)

85

Box 7.2 Peter Green – serial sex assault under sedation

In 1989 Peter Green developed a research proposal to study back pain. He advised his partners that he had received 2 years' funding from the University of Lough-borough, but continued into 1997. The project was designed for young adults but minors were also included. Green persuaded young men to undergo protracted and clinically unnecessary examinations while naked. Some of these examinations were illicitly video-recorded and some involved the use of injected sedation with the potential for retrograde amnesia. Between 1985 and 1997 a number of patients tried to raise concerns about their consultations with the Family Health Service Authority (FHSA), doctors at the practice, police and officers of the GMC. A health visitor raised concerns with the practice in 1996 and 1997. Green was stopped only in 1997, when the medical director of the Fosse Healthcare Community Trust contacted Leicestershire Health Authority to register concern, leading to Green's prosecution. While Green was expelled from the partnership, he continued to practise until his suspension in 1998. In 2000 he was finally convicted on nine counts of indecent assault on five patients.

Source: Commission for Health Improvement (2001).

Many recommendations were made, mostly relating to regulation of the medical profession and the aim was that 'the Inquiry will … seek to devise improved systems of control which will prevent such abuse in the future' (vol. 1, p. 107). One must fervently hope that such abuse, now we have a precedent, would never be so grossly overlooked or prolonged, though 'never again' is a hard goal in the real world.

Recent GMC cases

Boxes 7.2–7.5 illustrate the type and breadth of cases that the GMC is regularly called on to deal with.

Green's conviction (Box 7.2) was the culmination of concerns raised over 12 years and followed three separate police investigations. Files of evidence for the first two investigations, in 1985 and 1993, were submitted to the Crown Prosecution Service (CPS) but neither resulted in further action. The Secretary of State for Health invited the Commission for Health Improvement (CHI) to undertake an investigation. The resultant report found:

An NHS culture that did not listen to, or treat complaints inquisitively. The way in which NHS staff and patients related their experience to CHI described a system which allowed a credible person to do incredible things to patients to whom he had a duty of care. (Commission for Health Improvement, 2001)

The report describes a fudged and half-hearted way of dealing with complaints and concerns over many years, within both the practice and the local FHSA. This is perhaps best understood in the context of the finding that there was a belief within the partnership that other research undertaken by

Peter Green had been appropriate, for example research published previously in peer referenced journals. This may have led partners to be less probing than they might otherwise have been. The belief may also have been reinforced by Peter Green's style, which was described as imposing, articulate and authoritative.

The Tutin case (Box 7.3) illustrates how some GPs seem to be able to get away with patient abuse for many years without any effective intervention to stop them. It also shows that an abusive doctor may pose a threat to junior colleagues, and that both internal and external checks can fail.

Trust is an essential element of the doctor–patient relationship. GPs who abuse their patients therefore not only injure those they abuse but also injure the trust that other patients place in their own GPs. The Otterburn case (Box 7.4) illustrates that it is not only those directly involved with an offence who are affected.

A recent case (Box 7.5) illustrates that abuse is not always one way.

Box 7.3 Alan Tutin – sexual assault and inappropriate behaviours

Alan Tutin, from Guildford, was found guilty of misconduct by the GMC for sexually abusing five women between 1984 and 1999, and inappropriate behaviour in relation to another two patients, which continued up to 2006. Tutin also admitted using a telephone and a computer at the surgery to call sex lines and to access pornographic websites. The GMC found that Tutin made sexual advances towards a trainee GP who depended on him to sign off her training, and when she rebuffed him went further by telling her to take all her clothes off.

Source: GMC website (http://www.gmc-uk.org/), details of erasure, GMC no. 1729634.

Box 7.4 David Otterburn – possessor of child pornography

David Otterburn, from Abingdon, was prosecuted and found guilty of the possession of 100 images of child pornography and placed on the sex offenders' register. He was subsequently reported to the GMC, but initially sought voluntary erasure in order to avoid further penalty. He demonstrated a persistent lack of insight into the seriousness of his actions, notwithstanding regret and remorse reported in papers before the GMC panel.

A local paper recorded the views of former patients. One mother of three, whose family was treated for 25 years, said:

> I was told he had suddenly decided to take retirement which was long overdue. I was sick, absolutely disgusted, when I found out why he'd gone. My stomach just turned. People have been taking their children to see this man for years and he's been looking at indecent images of children.

Sources: Source: GMC website (http://www.gmc-uk.org/), details of erasure, GMC no. 1613511; http://www.heraldseries.co.uk/news/4167746.GP_cautioned_for_child_porn (accessed 18 September 2009).

Box 7.5 Lewis Dickinson – blackmailed for masturbating a patient

Dickinson had been blackmailed by a male patient whom he had masturbated, allegedly by mutual consent, during an examination. Dickinson allegedly paid the patient £100 weekly for over 2 years to buy his silence. When Dickinson stopped paying, the patient complained to the police. The patient was prosecuted by the police for blackmail, and Dickinson was reported to the GMC. His name was erased from the Medical Register in 2009.

Source: GMC website (http://www.gmc-uk.org/), details of erasure, GMC no. 2344577.

General lessons about patient abuse in general practice

Hafferty, in his chapter in the excellent book *Measuring Medical Professionalism*, states that 'all social groups need to celebrate their heroes and denounce their villains. … Groups also must establish their normative and moral boundaries' (Hafferty, 2006, p. 293).

There is much interest in assessing and even measuring medical professionalism. Conscientiousness can be measured, and trends have been shown to persist over time in UK medical students (Engel *et al*, 2009). Negative undergraduate student behaviour is associated with problems in a doctor's postgraduate career (McLachlan *et al*, 2009). In the USA, problematic students were more likely to be disciplined later as doctors by state disciplinary boards (Papadakis *et al*, 2004). The Green and Ayling cases illustrate the need for pattern recognition. An individual complaint requires a fair examination of the evidence, but surely repeated complaints must cause organisational alarm bells to ring? Yet the evidence suggests that we are not good at hearing such alarms.

It is right to be concerned about GPs who display behavioural characteristics such as arrogance, aloofness, an automatic rejection of criticism or a reluctance to address complaints. It is hoped that the current GMC proposals for revalidation via strengthened appraisal, including patient surveys and multi-source feedback from colleagues, will enable such traits to be addressed. This is, however, completely different from the fantasy that revalidation will always be effective as a way of stopping patient abuse. Had revalidation been in place it might have weeded out Ayling, but maybe not Green. Shipman would almost certainly have passed with flying colours, as his patients loved him and the dead do not complain.

In the Shipman report, Dame Janet Smith states 'I think it important for the future that all healthcare professionals recognise, as a duty, the fact that they should view the actions and performance of fellow professionals with independence of mind and professional objectivity' (vol. 5, p. 26). We must recognise, however, that there are inevitable barriers to the recognition, and therefore to the challenge, of deviant behaviour. The Ayling report recognised that GPs 'have little or no desire to judge a peer' (Paufley, 2004, p. 19) It is alarming to read that in 1998 only 47% of New Zealand GPs felt it should be mandatory to report doctor–patient sexual contact that came to their attention (White & Coverdale, 1998). Revalidation is set to use tools that are likely to prove too non-specific, with too high a rate of false positives and false negatives, to come to reliable conclusions about likely patient abuse. It may be reasonable to hope that revalidation will modestly reduce the likelihood of some of the worst instances of persistent patient abuse in general practice. However, it is surely wishful thinking to expect a full cure.

Conclusion

Sir William Osler (1932) said 'It is as important to know what kind of a man has the disease as it is to know what kind of a disease the man has'. Overlooking the gendered language, we might now add that 'It is as important to know what kind of a man is giving the treatment as it is to know what kind of treatment the man is giving'.

Surely the best hope of detecting the abuse of patients in general practice lies in a medical environment that listens to patients, takes complaints seriously, and forms a proper picture by joining up the dots. Such an environment takes pattern recognition seriously, and is prepared to ask unthinkable questions when the pattern demands. Years of delay in patient abuse coming to light still characterise some cases appearing before the GMC. It is too early to say whether GMC plans for revalidation of GPs via strengthened appraisal will change this. It is clear that there is no place for complacency.

References

Berlant, J. (1975) *Profession and Monopoly.* University of California Press.

Bristol Royal Infirmary Inquiry (2001) *Learning from Bristol: The Report of the Public Inquiry into Children's Heart Surgery at the Bristol Royal Infirmary 1984–1995* (Bristol Inquiry final report). Bristol Royal Infirmary Inquiry. Online at http://www.bristol-inquiry.org.uk/final_report/rpt_print.htm (accessed June 2010).

British Medical Association (2000) *Work Related Stress Among Senior Doctors.* BMA.

Caplan, R. (1994) Stress, anxiety and depression in hospital consultants, general practitioners and senior health service managers. *BMJ,* **309,** 1261–1263.

Commission of Health Improvement (2001) *Investigation into Issues Arising from the Case of Loughborough GP Peter Green.* TSO (The Stationery Office).

Emerson, Joan P. (1970) Behaviour in private places: sustaining definitions of reality in gynaecological examinations. In *Recent Sociology No. 2* (ed. H. Dreitzel), pp. 74–97. Macmillan.

Engel, N., Dmetrichuk, J. & Shanks, A. (2009) Medical professionalism: can it and should it be measured? *BMJ Careers,* **339,** 161.

Firth-Cozens, J. & Greenhalgh, J. (1997) Doctors' perceptions of the links between stress and lowered clinical care. *Social Science and Medicine*, **44**, 1017–1022.

Foucault, M. (1989) *The Birth of the Clinic*. Routledge. First published as *Naissance de la Clinique*. Presses Universitaires de France (1963).

Freidson, E. (1985) The reorganisation of the medical profession. *Medical Care Review*, **42**, 11–35.

Freudenberger, H. (1974) Staff burnout. *Journal of Social Issues*, **30**, 159–165.

General Medical Council (2004) *The Duties of a Doctor*. GMC. Available online at http://www.gmc-uk.org/guidance/good_medical_practice/duties_of_a_doctor.asp (accessed June 2010).

Hafferty, F. (2006) Measuring professionalism: a commentary. In *Measuring Medical Professionalism* (ed. D. Stern), pp. 281–306. Oxford University Press.

Illich, I. (1976) *Medical Nemesis: The Expropriation of Health*. Marion Boyars.

Jewson, N. (1976) Disappearance of the sick-man from medical cosmologies 1770–1870. *Sociology*, **10**, 225–244.

Kennedy, I. (1981) *The Unmasking of Medicine*. Allen and Unwin.

Lief, H. & Fox, R. (1963) Training for detached concern in medical students. In *The Psychological Basis of Medical Practice* (ed. H. Lief), pp. 12–35. Harper and Row.

McLachlan, J., Finn, G. & Macnaughton, J. (2009) The conscientiousness index: a novel tool to explore students' professionalism. *Academic Medicine*, **84**, 559–565.

McManus, I., Keeling, A. & Paice, E. (2004) Stress, burnout and doctors' attitudes to work are determined by personality and learning style. *BMC Medicine*, 2:29 doi:10.1186/1741-7015-2-29.

Misselbrook D. (2001) *Thinking About Patients*. Petroc (now Radcliffe).

Osler, W. (1932) *Aequanimitas* (3rd edition). Blakiston.

Papadakis, M., Hodgson, C., Teherani, A., *et al* (2004) Unprofessional behaviour in medical school is associated with subsequent disciplinary action by a state medical board. *Academic Medicine*, **79**, 244–249.

Paufley, A. (2004) *Committee of Inquiry: Independent Investigation into How the NHS Handled Allegations About the Conduct of Clifford Ayling*. Department of Health.

Schattner, P. (1998) Stress in general practice. How can GPs cope? *Australian Family Physician*, **27**, 993–998.

Shaw, G. B. (1911) *The Doctor's Dilemma*. Constable.

Smith, J. (2002) *The Shipman Enquiry*. HMSO.

Starr, P. (1982) *The Social Transformation of American Medicine*. Basic Books.

Tuckett, D., Boulton, M., Olson, C., *et al* (1985) *Meetings Between Experts*. Tavistock.

White, G. & Coverdale, J. (1998) General practitioner attitudes towards mandatory reporting of doctor–patient sexual abuse. *New Zealand Medical Journal*, **111**, 53–55.

Wilmshurst, P. (2000) Devaluing clinical skills. Personal view. *BMJ*, **320**, 1739.

CHAPTER 8

Boundaries and boundary violations in psychotherapy

Chess Denman

Overview

This chapter reviews actions which might represent boundary violations in psycho-therapy and looks at attempts to produce model guidelines for maintaining bound-aries. Risk factors which predispose to boundary violations are reviewed. Particular types of boundary violation are considered in turn with a psychotherapeutically informed perspective on why these may occur. The prevention of boundary viola-tions, their management and the treatment of patients are discussed. Finally, the chapter examines why certain writers have criticised aspects of the regulation of boundary violations in psychotherapy.

Introduction

Psychotherapists have had particular reasons for being interested in the preservation or loss of boundaries in their treatment interactions. Psychotherapy is an intimate activity, for the most part conducted privately, with little opportunity for direct oversight or social control. Yet it must maintain itself as a separate activity from other intimate interactions between pairs of individuals in order to be defined as a distinct social form. Thus psychotherapists are sensitive to charges that they are 'just offering friendship' or are comparable to prostitutes in offering intimate experiences paid on an hourly rate. Psychotherapy also brings a variety of different theories, all of which are relevant to the analysis of human relations and interactions. It is therefore not surprising that psychotherapists, especially psychodynamic psychotherapists, have developed a set of theoretical notions to apply to the analysis of professional relationships and their proper boundaries.

General boundaries

In general medical practice, the boundaries of ethical practice represent an extension of principles of criminal behaviour or civil damage (rape, fraud, etc.) to wider general notions of fiduciary duty and a duty of care. To an extent, this takes into account the idea that a medical professional may, by virtue of his or her position, be able to exert undue influence on a patient. This power should not be abused for personal or professional gain or exercised other than in the service of the patient's best interests and in a way which maintains the dignity and autonomy of the patient.

Boundaries in psychotherapy

In psychotherapy, and particularly psychodynamic psychotherapy, a stricter definition has been adopted, to include deviations from technical standards. These have featured injunctions to maintain high levels of analyst personal reticence and non-disclosure. While the techniques advocated may vary between different schools of therapy, most have adopted the principle that certain technical infractions represent boundary crossing or, worse, boundary violation.

Psychotherapists have tended to view the analysis of the reasons for the crossing of boundaries as more complex than a simple matter of ethical practice or action between two autonomous individuals. Psychodynamic psychotherapists, for example, see both therapist and patient as subject to unconscious forces which may motivate and influence their behaviour whatever their conscious attitude (Box 8.1). Furthermore, all therapies recognise that the individuals involved may well be less rational in their conscious appraisal of the situations because they are subject to disunities of will and of consciousness. The extent therefore to which the maintenance of proper boundaries, good professional practice and accurate psychotherapeutic technique can be consciously willed and enacted may be more limited than at first appears to be the case. Additionally, a concern with unconscious

---

Box 8.1 A therapist's unconscious motivation

A therapist was 5 minutes late for a session. The patient angrily complained and the therapist defended herself by saying that she was unavoidably detained. This caused the patient even more fury: 'I heard you gossiping with the secretary in the office next to the waiting room'. This was true. The therapist was forced to reflect on her anxieties about this patient (who often felt suicidally depressed) and her reason for avoiding contact.

---

motivation and a focus on the particular kinds of relationship which build up in longer-term psychotherapy have led therapists to argue that this potential for undue influence extends for a considerable period (possibly even forever) after the ending of formal treatment.

Psychotherapists have also extended the concept of boundaries in therapy by using the analysis of deviations (often termed 'enactments') from a standard frame of practice as a tool for investigating the unconscious processes both in the therapist and in the patient. This makes certain boundary crossing a sort of *felix culpa* (a fortunate sin) which may be turned to the good with careful handling.

The regulation of boundaries in psychotherapy

The intimate setting, the potential for undue influence and a range of high-profile cases of seriously exploitative behaviour by therapists have all led to the production of ethical guidelines for therapists now embodied in codes of practice. Almost all organisations which regulate or register psychotherapists publish ethical guidelines for appropriate practice which cover the possibility of boundary violations. The United Kingdom Council for Psychotherapy (UKCP) and the British Psychoanalytic Council have ethical guidelines (available on their respective websites, at http://www.psychotherapy. org.uk and http://www.psychoanalytic-council.org). However, the most comprehensive guidelines are published by the British Association for Counselling and Psychotherapy (BACP) (http://www.bacp.co.uk/ethical_ framework). These begin with a statement of values and then use the general ethical principles of *fidelity* to the trust placed in the practitioner, *honouring the autonomy* of the client, *acting with beneficence* towards the client and maintaining a stance of *non-maleficence* while seeking to do *justice* between competing demands and maintaining a level of self-respect. These principles go far beyond a simple concern to maintain certain minimum standards in psychotherapy and avoid boundary violations. The guidelines offer advice on maintaining a good quality of care, and state that practitioners should not attempt treatments beyond their competence. They should be clear about rights and responsibilities, avoid dual relationships and keep appropriate records. The 'Keeping trust' section covers confidentiality and explicitly condemns sexual activity with, or exploitation of, the client. In relation to financial or business relationships, the guidelines are less clears, advising that 'Practitioners should think carefully about, and exercise considerable caution before, entering into personal or business relationships with former clients and should expect to be professionally accountable if the relationship becomes detrimental to the client or the standing of the profession'.

Modern ethical guidelines have generally adopted the principle of framing recommendations in positive terms, telling therapists what they have a duty to do rather than refrain from. They are often short on examples

---

Box 8.2 Touching

A patient had completed a particularly challenging session of systematic desensitis-ation and had bravely handled a spider. The therapist patted her on the back but she flinched away in fright. The therapist noticed and asked what had been going through the patient's mind. The patient revealed that she had been the subject of unwanted advances by a previous therapist and was worried that her therapy would now take a sinister turn. The patient and therapist talked about sexual and non-sexual touching and the matter was resolved but the therapist made a note not to have physical contact with this patient in future.

---

of boundary violations. The guidelines produced by the Massachusetts Board of Regulation (cited in Hundert & Appelbaum, 1995) are helpful in this respect. They advise clear negotiation of fees and avoidance of the use of barter or any kind of collusion with the client to deceive insurers. They counsel the avoidance of economic relationships between therapist and patient, particularly those of employee–employer. The guidelines recommend care over physical contact, and suggest that while an appropriate physical examination in a medical context, a handshake or comforting pat in a public setting or in behavioural therapy might be appropriate, further contact is not (Box 8.2).

One difficulty with guidelines has been that different models of psycho-therapy have adopted a range of different standards of practice and taken different views about what constitutes an ethically appropriate relationship with the patient. There is agreement at the serious end of the spectrum (sexual and financial exploitation) but widespread disagreement in relation to less serious issues. Glass (2003) discusses this in relation principally to psychodynamic psychotherapy. He distinguishes between infractions which are distinct, discussable and non-progressive and those which are silent, sequential and could represent the beginning of a 'slippery slope' towards a more serious situation. This notion is helpful because it allows therapists to evaluate the moral context and emotional tone in which potential and actual boundary violations might occur.

Intimacy, sex and self-disclosure

Given the universal nature of sexual drives, it should be hardly surprising that among the many pairs of individuals who meet regularly to talk about intimate matters some will end up having sex. Nevertheless, there is general agreement that therapists are charged with avoiding this and with maintaining a stance of relative non-disclosure in relation to personal details, particularly in relation to sexual feelings towards the client. Indeed, there is some evidence that direct disclosure of sexual feelings by the therapist can trouble patients and precede more serious boundary violations (Fisher, 2004).

While there are well-documented cases of therapists who are serial sexual predators and actual sexual assault does occur, in these situations the agency of the therapist is easy to perceive. However, sexual activity in therapy may involve greater or lesser degrees of apparent consent or even initiative by the patient. After the event, just as in sustained sexual abuse in other situations, the victims may be troubled by reflections on whether they may have consented to or provoked the situation.

Different schools of psychotherapy have conceptualised the motivations behind pulls towards sexual intimacy in the psychotherapeutic situation in accord with their theoretical perspective. For psychoanalytically oriented psychotherapists, who argue both for the universality of sexual wishes and their primacy as a motivating force in human affairs, sexualisation of the therapeutic relationship always occurs, albeit in disguised form. Furthermore, they suggest that all relationships (and therapeutic relationships particularly) are contaminated with the memories and desires of past relationships. This phenomenon, termed 'transference', means that the therapist may at times be viewed not realistically but instead as though he or she were father, mother, a sibling or another important figure from the past. Thus wishes regarding the therapist, whether conscious or unconscious, are re-enlivenments of past wishes. Since in psychoanalytic theory unrequited sexual wishes regarding parents often represent a painful focus of emotional difficulty, the phenomenon of transference towards the therapist may also be highly sexual.

A less radical conception derives from attachment theory. Attachment is conceptualised as a biologically based system for ensuring affiliation and is particularly active in situations of dependency. While sexual urges are under the control of a separate system, there is clearly an activation of the attachment system during sexual attraction. Lovers' behaviour towards each other has close resemblances to mother–baby interactions. Since psychotherapy involves an offer of support and sympathy for someone in trouble, it frequently generates dependency, so attachment wishes, needs and regrets come to the fore. Attachment and sexual wishes are closely aligned for some patients, who may become erotically attracted to the therapist and become vulnerable to predatory therapists, in effect trading sex for attachment.

For other schools, such as cognitive–behavioural therapy and humanistic psychotherapy, theorisations of sexual activity and of the sexualisation of therapy are less complicated. In general, these schools have borrowed the notions of transference and undue influence without much consideration of the theoretical basis needed to incorporate these ideas.

Whatever differences attachment theorists and more traditional psychoanalytic theorists may have over the mechanism, both propose that the therapeutic situation has the potential to impair the autonomy and judgement of patients, so that their consent to sexual activity is never reliable. Thus it remains the duty of the therapist to take responsibility for refraining from sexual contact, irrespective of the wishes of the patient. Controversy continues only regarding the length of the period after the end of therapy for which this prohibition should endure. Some jurisdictions ban sexual activity in perpetuity. Others try to set time limits with caveats about cooling-off periods, further therapy for both parties, and rules about who may make initial contact. The central issue at stake is the believed duration of impaired autonomy following the ending of therapy.

Anger, abuse and assault

Earlier therapists concentrated on the loving impulses patients had towards their therapists and the loving and erotic wishes patients had towards their own parents. The later development of psychoanalytic and cognitive–behavioural theory (Beck, 1999) turned towards hatred and anger as important human motivations. Similarly, boundary violations by therapists may as easily be hating as eroticised: it is rare, but not unheard of, for therapists to assault patients physically (Masson, 1988). Verbal abuse and abuse of power are more common. Little acts of anger are commonplace, such as deliberately starting a session late or refusing to offer a basic level of human sympathy when clearly warranted.

Why do these infractions occur? Many of the patients with whom therapists work are trapped in ill-serving interpersonal interactions, such as evoking angry, frustrated or hating responses from others. Therapists, too, may respond with anger but should explore ways to relate to such individuals in order to help them to change those patterns. Sadly, not all hating results solely from such potentially remedial responses. For some therapists, patients who are insufficiently admiring or grateful or who do not recover under their care become frustrating and hateful. The therapist may respond with smaller or larger acts of anger, as in Box 8.3, but curbing

---

Box 8.3 A suicidal threat

A patient telephoned his therapist late on a Friday afternoon. He said he was suicidal and was standing at a railway station thinking of jumping in front of a train. He challenged the therapist to 'do something about it'. This was one of many such telephone calls. Generally the therapist responded sympathetically, trying to explore reasons for the sudden increase in suicidal feelings and to help the patient plan activities. This time the therapist found himself saying 'Well, if the trains are going slowly as they leave the station you might not come to much harm.' The patient slammed the telephone down. The therapist had an anxious weekend and was very relieved to see the patient still alive and well at their next session.

---

a frustrated or hating response in order to analyse and 'metabolise' it is a central therapeutic skill.

This sort of boundary violation can lead to guilt on the part of the therapist, who may take some reparative action such as extending a session, but feel unconsciously resentful of the demand. This may fuel a more serious error, such as forgetting to tell the patient about an upcoming holiday break. The fury expressed subsequently by the patient now drives the therapist to make more inappropriate concessions. Out of such oscillating cycles increasingly serious boundary violations can develop.

Abuse of the patient for dependency needs

Erotic and hating motivations are not the only ones which drive therapists and patients. Ever since the work of Bowlby (1991), the power of needs deriving from dependency attachment and affiliation has been recognised. Some therapists exploit the therapeutic situation to meet their own attachment needs. They come to depend on the love and support of their patients and begin to violate the boundaries of therapy by increasing self-disclosure of their own difficulties.

Financial impropriety and gifts

In private settings, patients are entitled to a clear negotiation of fees to be charged and their treatment should not be unnecessarily prolonged. Patients treated in the state system are entitled to a fair and just distribution of often limited resources. Therapists may collude in not letting patients know that funding scarcity is the reason that they have been denied treatment or are being offered only limited treatment, perhaps provided by a student therapist.

Patients often bring gifts. Therapists from different schools have treated this situation differently: some refuse to accept all gifts, while more commonly others accept small gifts at appropriate times, for instance at Christmas or the ending of treatment. However, it is worth bearing in mind that the size of a gift may seem very different to an impoverished patient and to a middle-class therapist, and that gifts may have different meanings for patients at different times.

Dual relationships and conflicts of interest

If patients are to be able to express their hopes and fears freely, then their therapist must not have a hold over them in other areas. Therapists who are also employers or supervisors, or who otherwise have power over the patient in the external world, are unlikely to be able to pretend not to know either what has occurred in treatment or what is occurring in the outer world. For this reason therapists should avoid 'dual relationships'.

Confidentiality and case reports

There has been enduring concern with issues of confidentiality. Therapists have tended to see themselves as protectors of the patient's interests against the requirements of the state or other organisations (Bolas & Sundelson, 1996). It is generally accepted now that a duty of confidentiality towards the patient is not absolute. For instance, the duty to report any serious worry about 'significant harm' coming to a child is enshrined in the Children Act 1989. A number of legal jurisdictions impose a duty on practitioners to breach confidentiality in situations where a significant risk exists to another person, following the ruling in *Tarasoff* v. *Regents of the University of California* (1976; see http://www.publichealthlaw.net/Reader/docs/Tarasoff.pdf).

Therapists have been slower to identify their own breaches of confidentiality. Only recently has the risk of patients identifying themselves in relation to case reports been appreciated. Psychotherapeutic literature has depended to a great extent on case reports, both as sources of evidence and as illustrative examples. Arguably, only reports which are so disguised as to count as fiction are ethically acceptable, unless the patient consents (Denman, 2003).

Risk factors for sexual boundary violation

It seems reasonable to suppose that risk factors vary between different types of boundary violator. Gabbard & Lester (2003) produces a typology of sexual boundary violators. Three groups – predatory psychopaths (Box 8.4), those with a paraphilia (sexual deviation) and psychotic therapists – have evident pathology. They seem very different from those he classifies as 'love-sick' – lonely therapists with relationship difficulties who seek fulfilment in a relationship with a patient with whom they believe they are genuinely in love. A second, less pathological group, whose motivation is characterised as 'masochistic surrender', are therapists who persuade themselves that sexual contact is in the service of therapy. Further work is needed, particularly on predatory psychopaths. They are rare but may account for a disproportionately high number of cases because of the large number of victims. Methods which allow reliable early identification of such therapists and their exclusion from professional practice should be a research priority.

In the group of therapists whose boundary violations are isolated deviations from practice there is general agreement that loneliness and social isolation are predisposing factors (Norris *et al*, 2003).

Box 8.4 The predatory psychopath

A patient revealed she had been sexually exploited by a previous therapist. He had sexually assaulted her during a therapy session and then announced that because she had significant mental health problems her story would not be believed. She did not act until she saw in the local paper that the therapist had been disciplined for a sexual assault on another patient. When she came forward to tell her story she found that other women had also found the courage to come forward. There was some comfort in finding that she was not alone. However, the perpetrator stoutly denied all impropriety and maintained contemptuously that the women involved were in the grip of a collective delusion.

Not all patients are equally at risk. Norris *et al* (2003) discuss factors that exacerbate the vulnerability of patients: those who are dependent on the therapist or whose reason for seeking therapy is partly to experience an intense relationship are at risk, as are those whose prior experience of abuse has conditioned them to expect abusive therapy relationships and disabled their capacity to question their experiences. Ben-Ari & Somer (2004) reviewed 14 female victims of abuse and characterised them as 'problem saturated' and lonely. Many had a history of sexual abuse. This group is vulnerable to sexual exploitation generally, so it is doubly tragic when they are abused in therapy.

Not all therapies are of equal risk, although serious boundary violations have occurred in all kinds of practice. General features, such as the length of the therapy (long), the setting (the therapist's home) and the degree of oversight (low) are probably the most important features of risky therapies. Paradoxically, senior therapists practise in a particularly risky way: they more often conduct long therapies with more seriously disturbed and consequently vulnerable patients, either in an isolated institutional setting or in private practice, and may be subject to less oversight. Junior therapists may be less risky: they are usually supervised and conduct therapies whose duration is planned and limited.

Effects of boundary crossing and boundary violation

Opinion is divided on the extent to which boundary crossings are inevitable and the therapeutic use which can be made of them. The idea that cycles of rupture and repair in the therapeutic alliance (Safran *et al*, 2001) are part of the therapeutic process is widespread and accounts for the idea that boundary crossing may be therapeutic if handled right.

Once abuse and boundary violation have occurred, all are agreed that patients are likely to suffer harm. Luepker (1999) looked at 55 women who had been sexually abused in therapy. Many described an increase in symptoms of post-traumatic stress disorder (PTSD), with lowered mood. Alcohol and drug use increased and the women reported relationship or work problems. Even more worryingly, the women reported that they found it hard to get help and 18% were sexually revictimised in subsequent treatments. There is some evidence that the context of the abuse determines the degree of damage done and its nature. Somer & Nachmani (2005) were able to distinguish 'romantic' and 'abusive' narratives in their patients' accounts of sexual boundary violations. They found that those who had romantic accounts were less damaged, but cautioned that both groups of exploited women showed impairment on measures of psychiatric health.

The mechanism by which non-consensual sex, rape or violent abuse in therapy causes harm is likely to be little different from that operating after other sexual assaults. Patients will be likely to suffer adjustment reactions and a proportion will develop PTSD symptoms. For those to whom the experience seems more consensual, the psychodynamics are likely to resemble those where patients are pressed into sex of a taboo nature, such as incest. It is not surprising that survivor shame (Penfold, 1999) is a significant factor. These patients ask themselves why they kept attending therapy. They may feel that they were complicit in the experience and so feel contaminated, with significant lowering of self-esteem.

Prevention

Prevention involves the management of risk factors. Therapists at greater risk of boundary violation should be identified as far as possible and either excluded from the profession or tightly supervised. Situations which predispose to boundary violations should be closely managed. Therapists, especially the most senior, should avoid long hours of isolated practice without regular supervision and oversight. Self-monitoring by the profession involves helping therapists to identify early warning signs. The ideas of a slippery slope or a natural history of misconduct (Simon, 1999) can be helpful. Therapists can monitor therapy for signs of drift into dangerous territory. Epstein & Simon (1990) have developed an 'Exploitation Index', which therapists can use to monitor themselves for potential infractions.

The training and continuing professional development of therapists need to include a prominent educational component directed at boundary violation. It is helpful to involve patients brave enough to share their experiences. Continuing supervision is essential. However, a powerful force which can render both educational and supervisory inputs futile is the feeling that develops in therapists that their particular boundary violation is in some way exceptional or special and therefore exempt from the rules. More than any other, this feature of perceived specialness needs to be highlighted in education and supervision.

Treating patients who have experienced boundary violations

Once serious boundary violations are known or suspected, the key principles to guide immediate action are patient safety and well-being. Therapists who become aware of or who suspect boundary violations by colleagues need to be prepared to take prompt and effective action. Sadly, the history of many high-profile cases involving serious sexual assaults reveals that this often does not occur. Some patients may be willing to make a formal complaint; others do not feel strong enough. The safety of other patients means that professionals who come to know about boundary violations by therapists have a duty to act on this knowledge and to initiate investigations and appropriate action.

Patients who do make complaints are likely to need support, especially if they have to recount personal and distressing experiences. Every effort should be made to avoid repetition of this, as can happen particularly when a range of regulatory authorities act individually and often in sequence to discipline the therapist. While bringing perpetrators to justice is a healing process for some patients, others may be re-traumatised by the repeated retelling of their tale, particularly those with significant PTSD symptoms. Professionals should offer support but not assume that they are the best people to do so. Support groups for victims of abuse in therapy may be equally or more helpful.

Unfortunately, the simple guarantee that patients who have experienced boundary violations can expect to receive the same standard of care that all patients should expect is often hard to make good. As with all traumatic or distressing experiences, patients will have a range of reactions. Some will not wish for nor need further treatment and it should not be pressed on them; others will experience substantial symptoms and may suffer from enduring ill effects.

Patients who want continuing professional help should be assessed by a professional who has training and expertise in this area. It may be appropriate to offer further therapy in the same or different modality or to consider the use of psychotropic medication. Patients whose trust in psychiatry, psychology or therapy has been badly damaged can be helped by a frank and open discussion with an independent expert. Every effort should be made to treat the patient in an organisation which is both physically and bureaucratically separate from that in which the abuse took place. Therapy should help the patient to set the events in context and to overcome their effects. Patients often derive benefit from sharing their experiences with others in a similar situation and from knowing that they are not alone. Psycho-education and linking the patient up with local user groups or a national organisation should be prominent features of most treatments.

The ill effects of boundary violations do not end with the damage done to the patient and the therapist but extend to therapy itself. High-profile cases of boundary violation weaken public trust in therapists and therapy and may deter patients who could benefit from seeking help.

Reservations

Samuels (1999) argues that some therapists and regulatory organisations have become so mesmerised by boundary violations that they have forced therapists into a defensive position. This view is echoed by Kroll (2001), who worries that some of the guidelines that have been introduced – particularly those designed to prevent therapists from starting down a slippery slope – are too restrictive and may result in ossification of practice. Gutheil & Gabbard (1998) concur and suggest that at times a 'boundary panic' may occur, resulting in hasty or ill-considered action. The common finding that patients who have experienced significant boundary violations can have considerable difficulty in accessing further treatment is possibly a consequence of the anxieties that therapists have developed in this area.

Conclusion

Changes in the social context of medical and psychological treatment have emphasised patient choice and autonomy. Professionals are now held to account for their actions and infractions more systematically than before. It is hoped that this will reduce the incidence of boundary violations and consequent damage to patients. However, the nature of therapy and the ubiquity of the motives that drive unethical practice mean that such events are unlikely to be completely eliminated. A social, psychological and ethical understanding of boundary violations is critical to reducing their incidence and managing the aftermath when they do occur.

References

Beck, A. T. (1999) *Prisoners of Hate: The Cognitive basis of Anger, Hatred and Violence.* Harper-Collins.

Ben-Ari, A. & Somer, E. (2004) The aftermath of therapist–client sex: exploited women struggle with the consequences. *Clinical Psychology and Psychotherapy*, **11**, 126–136.

Bolas, C. & Sundelson, D. (1996) *The New Informants: The Betrayal of Confidentiality in Psychoanalysis and Psychotherapy.* Jason Aronson.

Bowlby, J. (1991) *Attachment and Loss. Vol. 3: Loss – Sadness and Depression.* Penguin Books.

Broden, M. S. (1999) Factors influencing psychologists' perceptions of clients who claim therapist sexual abuse: client incest history and psychologist gender. *Dissertation Abstracts International: Section B: The Sciences and Engineering*, vol. 60, no. 2–B, p. 0820.

Denman, C. (2003) *Sexuality: A Biopsychosocial Approach.* Palgrave Macmillan.

Epstein, R. S. & Simon, R. (1990) The Exploitation Index: an early warning indicator of boundary violations in psychotherapy. *Bulletin of the Menninger Clinic*, **54**, 450–465.

Fisher, C. D. (2004) Ethical issues in therapy: therapist self-disclosure of sexual feelings. *Ethics and Behavior (Special Issue: Ethics and Behavior)*, **14**, 105–121.

Gabbard, G. O. & Lester, E. P. (2003) *Boundaries and Boundary Violations in Psychoanalysis*. American Psychiatric Publishing.

Glass, L. L. (2003) The gray areas of boundary crossings and violations. *American Journal of Psychotherapy*, **57**, 429.

Gutheil, T. G. & Gabbard, G. O. (1998) Misuses and misunderstandings of boundary theory in clinical and regulatory settings. *American Journal of Psychiatry*, **155**, 409–414.

Hundert, E. M. & Appelbaum, P. S. (1995) Boundaries in psychotherapy: model guidelines. *Psychiatry: Interpersonal and Biological Processes*, **58**, 345–356.

Kroll, J. (2001) Boundary violations: a culture-bound syndrome. *Journal of the American Academy of Psychiatry and the Law*, **29**, 274–283.

Luepker, E. T. (1999) Effects of practitioners' sexual misconduct: a follow-up study. *Journal of the American Academy of Psychiatry and the Law*, **27**, 51–63.

Masson, J. M. (1988) *Against Therapy: Emotional Tyranny and the Myth of Psychological Healing*. Athenaeum Press.

Norris, D. M., Gutheil, T. G. & Strasburger, L. H. (2003) This couldn't happen to me: boundary problems and sexual misconduct in the psychotherapy relationship. *Psychiatric Services*, **54**, 517–522.

Penfold, S. P. (1999) Why did you keep going for so long? Issues for survivors of long-term, sexually abusive 'helping' relationships. *Journal of Sex Education and Therapy*, **24**, 244–251.

Safran, J. D., Muran, J. C., Samstag, L. W., *et al* (2001) Repairing alliance ruptures. *Psychotherapy: Theory, Research, Practice, Training*, **38**, 406–412.

Samuels, A. (1999) From sexual misconduct to social justice. Erotic transference and countertransference. In *Clinical Practice in Psychotherapy* (ed. D. Mann), pp. 150–171. Taylor & Francis/Routledge.

Simon, R. I. (1999) Therapist–patient sex: from boundary violations to sexual misconduct. *Psychiatric Clinics of North America*, **22**, 31–47.

Somer, E. & Nachmani, I. (2005) Constructions of therapist–client sex: a comparative analysis of retrospective victim reports. *Sexual Abuse: Journal of Research and Treatment*, **17**, 47–62.

CHAPTER 9

Sexual therapies: ethical guidelines, vulnerabilities and boundaries

Michael Crowe

Overview

The field of sexual therapy, because of the explicit content of what is discussed, is one in which the possibilities for sexual boundary breaking between therapist and client or patient are in theory quite high. However, there are a number of safeguards in place, including codes of ethics and practice, the insistence on supervision and the use of chaperones for physical examination. In the UK the incidence of boundary violations in this field seems to be low.

Introduction

Sexual problems and their management require a particular sensitivity in the therapist because the subject matter of the discourse between the client (or patient) and the therapist (or doctor) is the intimate sexual interaction of two people. The areas being discussed are rarely if ever spoken about in a serious way outside the intimate relationship itself. In some types of therapy a physical examination also has to take place. Here, too, sensitivity has to be exercised to avoid embarrassment and to put the patient at his or her ease while the examination is taking place or the devices to restore function are being demonstrated.

Background

The earliest form of sexual therapy in the UK was carried out at the Institute of Psychosexual Medicine (Tunnadine, 1970). The therapists were predominantly general medical practitioners trained by the psychodynamically oriented Dr Michael Balint. He used a 'seminar' method, in which groups of doctors met together with a supervisor. Many of the patients, and most of the doctors, were female, and the doctors were encouraged to carry out a vaginal examination, which could produce a 'moment of truth' in which the patient would reveal the reasons behind her presenting sexual problem. The method is still practised, but only in a minority of settings.

The foundations of sexual therapy as most widely practised today were put in place by Masters & Johnson (1970), who instituted the concept of the couple as the 'unit' for treatment, and used a combination of face-to-face meetings between the couple and two 'co-therapists' with homework exercises for the couple. Masters & Johnson used a rather unusual approach in which the couple stayed at a hotel in the city where the therapy took place, and attended the clinic every day for 2 weeks. Their methods have been imitated in many different settings, but in most of these the couples have attended once or twice a week at a clinic within travelling distance from their home address.

Sexual therapy takes many different forms, and there are many different professionals involved in the field. Those who work in sexual dysfunction using a psychosexual approach include psychiatrists, psychologists, nurses and counsellors, most of whom have had specific training in this work, and many of whom are accredited members of the British Association for Sexual and Relationship Therapy (BASRT; http://www.basrt.org.uk). They may work in National Health Service (NHS) settings such as psychiatric out-patient departments or genito-urinary medicine clinics, within Relate (originally the National Marriage Council, founded in 1938) or in private practice. They carry out psychosexual therapy with individuals and with couples. This involves an analysis of the sexual problems presented, an attempt to understand their psychological and physical causes, and therapeutic techniques based largely on 'homework exercises' to help the individual or couple to restore sexual function to an acceptable level. It is not usual for these practitioners to carry out physical examinations or physiological investigations, although in some cases they may be needed. A referral to a general practitioner (GP) or to a hospital urology or gynaecology department is the typical way of organising them.

In their work with couples, psychosexual therapists have to consider the relationship of the two partners as well as the sexual history and sexual attitudes of the individuals. Much of the therapy consists of trying to achieve an improvement in the couple's communication patterns and to alter unhelpful kinds of interaction which might be inhibiting the sexual life of the partnership (Crowe & Ridley, 2000: p. 294). In their work with individuals they tend to concentrate on helping to reduce anxiety about sexual functioning and to achieve a greater confidence in sexual performance.

Psychosexual therapists may also help patients who have related problems, such as transvestism, gender dysphoria and sexual addiction. Here the focus is almost always on the individual, even though the problem may indirectly influence the patient's relationship as well as his or her own well-being.

There are other professionals who deal with sexual problems using a more physically based approach. For example, there is a service for erectile problems in the urology department of many general hospitals. Here the surgeons investigate the problems, with an emphasis on physiological investigations such as penile blood flow assessment and penile plethysmography. The management of the patients is predominantly by physical intervention, the most frequent method being the prescription of phosphodiesterase inhibitors such as sildenafil (Viagra), or the demonstration and prescription of vacuum pumps for the creation of an erection by drawing blood into the corpora cavernosa. The prescription of medication is usually done by the surgeons in charge. The demonstration of the use of pumps, however, is usually carried out by urological nurses, who will often be members of the British Association of Urological Nurses (http://www.baun.co.uk), and there is necessarily physical contact between the treating professional and the patient. The nurses will often also enquire about psychological factors, and may offer a brief version of psychosexual therapy in addition to the physical methods.

In family planning clinics it is quite common for patients to complain of sexual dysfunctions, and the doctors and nurses in these settings build up a good deal of experience and expertise in helping them. The Royal College of Obstetricians and Gynaecologists has a Faculty for Sexual and Reproductive Health, to which many of those involved in family planning are affiliated. In the clinics themselves the main remit is naturally the management of contraception, although many women who attend also have sexual problems. The treatment of vaginismus and vulvodynia is often carried out by gynaecologists or those working with them, including family planning nurses, and often there are counsellors attached to the clinics who deal with other problems in the psychosexual field, such as low sexual desire or anorgasmia. Again, physical examination and physical contact between treating professional and patient is the usual practice.

Ethical issues in sexual therapies

The ethical difficulties posed by these approaches to sexual problems have not been fully researched. Those who engage in psychosexual work with patients are in constant discussion about sexual matters with them, whether they are seeing them as individuals or couples, and they clearly have to gather a large amount of confidential information. This puts them in a position of some trust, as well as giving them considerable power over the clients. There is a well-tried 'Code of Ethics and Principles of Good Practice for Members' published by the BASRT (and available on its website at http://www.basrt.org.uk/pdf/documents/6_code_ethics_members.pdf), which addresses the issues of maintenance of both ethical boundaries and confidentiality in this type of therapy (see below).

The clinical problems presented to psychosexual therapists often have ethical implications. For example, a therapist might be told of an affair by one member of a couple that the partner does not know about. If the couple are in therapy together this may cause a dilemma for the therapist as to how to deal with the information. The usual arrangement is to have an explicit discussion in advance (at the beginning of therapy) to inform both partners that what is disclosed in an individual session is confidential; but the therapist will often encourage the partner who has disclosed the affair to tell their partner about it, if this can be done without too much disruption.

A client may disclose a history of being the victim of child sexual abuse, and again the therapist has the dilemma of whether to take action in reporting this to the authorities, with the consent of the client. The general rule is that if the therapist considers that future harm may be prevented by doing so, then it would be right to report the allegation. Similarly, the disclosure of partner abuse during therapy would lead to the duty to report this if future harm can be avoided. Another common dilemma is the wish by distressed parents that the therapist should 'cure' their teenage son of his homosexuality. The usual advice, to let the young person make his own decision, is often met with a hostile response on the part of the parents.

There is another, related, ethical issue which is not relevant to anyone doing conventional sexual therapy, but which has caused difficulties for the BASRT in framing its rules. This is the question of 'surrogate therapy' for sexual dysfunctions. Masters & Johnson (1970) reported the use of both male and female surrogate partners for the treatment of clients who were unattached but wished to solve their sexual problems by the therapy offered by them. They employed sexually experienced men and women to help the clients to achieve successful intercourse, and the client and surrogate would become a temporary 'couple' for the duration of the therapy, going through the programme of conjoint meetings and hotel-based homework exercises just like an established couple. They reported that some of these single clients had good results from the therapy, but they gave up the practice in later years, partly because of difficulties in recruiting suitable surrogate partners. Surrogate therapy continues in various centres both in the USA and the UK, but it is very much separate from the mainstream of sexual therapy. The ethical problems involved are manifold, and the question of the clients effectively paying for sex with a surrogate partner has not been clarified legally. Indeed, the BASRT website specifically states that it does not recognise surrogate sexual therapy as legitimate.

Even leaving the question of surrogate therapy aside, the process of psychosexual therapy is full of ethical problems for the therapist. Some of the more difficult involve the sexual feelings of the therapist. It is impossible to carry out sexual therapy without discussing sexual function and sexual feelings in a very detailed way. In some cases it is difficult for the therapist to remain unaffected by the situation, particularly those therapists who are younger or more inexperienced. The advice that is usually given in training is that, in order to maintain some distance and objectivity, it is better to avoid the common terms for sexual organs or sexual activities, but instead to use the proper anatomical and physiological ones. It is also inadvisable to be light-hearted when speaking about sexual matters. The use of self-disclosure by the therapist is discouraged. The therapists must all have supervision by a senior practitioner, and if sexual feelings are aroused in therapy this should be discussed with the supervisor and recorded. If there is no way of dealing with the problem for the individual therapist, then another therapist might be asked to take over the case.

Codes of ethics and practice

It is in the psychosexual field (as opposed to urology or gynaecology settings) that the greatest prominence has been given to ethical issues. The BASRT has had its 'Code of Ethics and Principles of Good Practice for Members ' for the past 20 years or more, and this is clear about the need for respect for the individual client, and the dangers of exploitation of the relationship in any way, whether financially, socially or sexually. There are sanctions laid down for any infringements, which mainly involve suspension or cancellation of membership of the Association. The BASRT insists that all therapists who have accreditation, however senior or experienced, should be under regular supervision with an accredited supervisor, and this is considered useful protection against the possibility of unintended breaches of boundaries during therapy. It is, of course, recognised that even the most assiduous supervision cannot restrain the 'rogue' practitioner, who might be exploiting the relationship with clients and simply lying to the supervisor; however, in the case of most therapists this supervision provides sufficient protection to guard against unintentional slippage and the intrusion of unethical practices into a therapeutic relationship.

The BASRT is a small organisation, with a membership of about 750. It has a well-established complaints procedure, which is accepted by the UK Council for Psychotherapy, to which the BASRT is affiliated. The BASRT has received no complaints from clients of sexual impropriety in the past 6 years. Of the handful of other types of complaint, only one was upheld. Whether this absence of ethical boundary violations is simply a statistical anomaly because of the small size of the organisation, or whether the reason is that, from its outset, the BASRT has had high ethical standards, is not clear. It may also be related to the predominantly female membership. Whatever the reason, and in spite of the sexual content of much of the discussion that goes on in therapy, there seems to be a relatively low risk of violations among members of the Association.

The role of managers and senior practitioners is also important in reducing the risks of unethical practices within clinics. If it is the accepted rule that chaperones are always used in physical examinations, and that the dignity and modesty of the patients are respected at all times, then there is less risk of exploitation, whether intended or unintended, by staff.

The former client and dual relationships

There is at present no national consensus on whether, after the end of any psychotherapy, there should be a ban on other forms of relationship between the therapist and client. However, the Code of Ethics and Principles of Good Practice of the BASRT explicitly forbids such a change of relationship indefinitely. The full text can be accessed on the BASRT website. Some clauses may be usefully quoted here:

Code of Ethics: 2. The member is responsible to the client, for making and maintaining appropriate boundaries to the therapeutic relationship, both during and after therapy.

Principles of Good Practice: 21. The therapist has an ethical responsibility to act in the best interests of the client, be they present or past clients. The therapist must seek to avoid sexual, financial, emotional or any other form of client exploitation at all times.

Principles of Good Practice: 27. It is not acceptable for a therapist to engage in sexual contact or sexualised behaviour with anyone who is or has been his or her own sexual therapy client.

There are many other aspects of therapy, supervision and training which are covered by the BASRT Code of Ethics and Principles of Good Practice, and similar boundaries have to be maintained within all these types of relationship. For example, the supervisor is responsible for setting and maintaining the boundaries between the supervision relationship and other professional relationships, such as training or management (i.e. not having the trainee in both supervision and training at the same time). Similarly, a trainer should not have a training responsibility and a therapy or counselling contract with the same trainee over the same period of time. These are examples of 'dual relationships'.

Use of chaperones

For those who work in clinics where there is physical examination of the patients the issue is a different one, although they also have to ask about very intimate sexual matters. With physical examinations, practitioners have to exercise great caution in maintaining proper boundaries between themselves and the client. This will include the use of chaperones, and an explanation of what will be happening before each procedure is carried out. It is not clear whether all clinics use chaperones all the time, and in a busy clinic corners might be cut, especially in the case of patient and therapist being of the same gender.

Most of the nurses and other practitioners in clinics where physical examinations are carried out do not belong to the BASRT. However, the BASRT

Code of Ethics and Principles of Good Practice has some clauses which are relevant to their work, and it might be useful for those who work in this way to be aware of the Code. For example, in relation to physical procedures and chaperones it states:

Principles of Good Practice: 24. Consideration should be given to adequate chaperone cover when procedures involving physical contact are to be embarked upon.

Principles of Good Practice: 25. Therapeutic procedures involving physical contact must only be performed by someone specifically trained for such procedures.

Principles of Good Practice: 26. Physical examination to exclude organic disease must only be performed by a medical practitioner currently registered by the General Medical Council, unless the examination involves the pelvic region only and is carried out by someone specifically trained and qualified for this procedure, working under medical supervision.

It is not known exactly how many of the clinics involved in this work adhere to the recommendations on the use of chaperones, but it is likely that most of them follow the other recommendations in the code in relation to the need for training of those carrying out therapy involving the use of vacuum pumps and other devices. The involvement of these practitioners with patients is usually quite brief, and the risks of an inappropriate relationship developing are probably less than in the more intensive and longer-term forms of psychosexual therapy.

An illustrative case

There is an ever-present risk of unethical practice in sexual therapy, as in other forms of psychological and physical therapy, and in some cases the boundaries have been broken. Probably the best-documented case of sexual assault under the guise of therapy is that of a consultant psychiatrist, Michael Haslam (Box 9.1; see also Box 6.1, p. 65, on Haslam), who persuaded his female patients to undress in his presence in a remote part of the hospital and sexually assaulted them in the name of therapy (Department of Health, 2005).

In general there seem to be few cases in which a therapist has set out to seduce patients. In many cases, however, there has been some kind of mutual attraction between therapist and client which the therapist ought to have discouraged, but did not do so, and this might have resulted in an inappropriate relationship arising. The relationship may not at first have been sexual, but any relaxation of the boundaries, such as flirtatious comments, social invitations, therapist self-disclosure or offers for help in other aspects of life, can lead to a dangerous blurring of the differences between therapy and other types of relationship. To prevent this, the inculcation in therapy trainees of a respect for the therapeutic boundaries, along with the insistence

---

Box 9.1 Michael Haslam as psychosexual therapist

Michael Haslam, the consultant psychiatrist in York who was one of the subjects of the Kerr/Haslam Inquiry (Department of Health, 2005), also practised psychosexual therapy and claimed specialist expertise in this field. He was a non-accredited member of the BASRT, from which he subsequently resigned. His patients were not generally suffering from sexual problems, but he offered many of them massage to the body (supposedly designed to reduce anxiety and tension) with the patient unclothed and without a chaperone. He also took some of the patients to a remote part of the hospital in the name of research into a form of heat-sensitive photography of the hands (to detect levels of anxiety). Haslam was later convicted on four counts of indecent assault.

---

that they have supervision while carrying out therapy, may go some way towards reducing the risk of abuse of the relationship in this way.

Methods of avoiding the inappropriate crossing of boundaries

Training and codes

There are a number of courses in the UK for the training of psycho-sexual therapists, and on all of these the importance of an ethical code is emphasised. The trainees are taught the basics of ethical practice and are introduced to the BASRT Code of Ethics and Principles of Good Practice. It is not so clear how urology and family planning therapists are trained, and this remains an area where there may be some concern about ethical standards. However, the work in those settings is usually based on the use of teams, in contrast to psychosexual work, which is done in a consulting room with supervision provided after the event. It would, however, be useful to extend the use of ethical codes throughout the field of sexual treatment.

Supervision

The supervisor has a key role in monitoring the work of the therapist. Sessions are reported on a regular basis, and however senior the practitioner, there is an insistence by the BASRT that regular supervision takes place. Indeed, in order to achieve annual re-accreditation (and therefore continue practising under the Association) all practitioners need to obtain the signature of their supervisor to confirm that they have attended regularly. Supervision is not a panacea, and a rogue practitioner might get away with seducing patients by simply lying about it to the supervisor. However, these cases are hopefully rare. A less determined therapist who breaks boundaries might be suspected by the supervisor, who is trained to spot inconsistencies and act upon them.

Regulation

As mentioned above, many psychosexual therapists belong to the BASRT, and via that organisation have affiliation to the UK Council for Psychotherapy (UKCP; www.ukcp.org.uk). If therapists are also medical practitioners, psychologists, nurses or counsellors, they may also be affiliated to their own professional bodies. These bodies usually have a fully functional complaints procedure, which would take account of any infringement of the professional relationship between therapist and client and deal with it by sanctions. It is still, however, possible at present to call oneself a therapist without any professional affiliation at all. If a therapist chose to work in that way there is nothing to protect the client from an inappropriate relationship with the therapist. There is thus a theoretical risk that a registered therapist who had been accused of an infringement of the therapeutic relationship could resign from the regulatory body and yet continue doing therapy. This may, however, be obviated if the professions of psychotherapy and counselling are subjected to statutory registration, which is at present expected to happen under the aegis of the Health Professions Council. In that event, it would be against the law to designate oneself as a therapist or counsellor without being registered under the Council.

Management

In settings such as the NHS there is a complaints procedure which most patients are aware of, and access to it has been facilitated in recent years, partly as a result of various scandals. Similarly, in Relate offices, where much psychosexual therapy takes place, the principles of supervision and oversight are well respected. In private practice, however, there is often no team and no colleagues, and the practitioner has to rely on the help of a supervisor (if the practitioner is in supervision) or simple self-regulation to guard against boundary violation. If the professions of psychotherapy and counselling are subject to registration under the Health Professions Council, all therapists and counsellors will have to be registered, and the need for supervision is emphasised in the codes of most organisations affiliated to the UKCP and the British Association for Counselling and Psychotherapy (BACP), whose practitioners would then be registered under the Council.

Conclusion

The field of sexual therapies is a wide and varied one, and there is no clear single solution to the problem of boundary violation. Sexual therapies necessarily involve the discussion of sexual history, of the sexual practices engaged in by the couple or individual, sexual fears and sexual fantasies, and in some settings physical examination. It is understandable that the therapist and the client are subject to pressures which, if they are not countered, may lead to an inappropriate involvement of the therapist with the client. This may simply take the form of the therapist becoming sexually attracted to the client, and this can be successfully dealt with if it is discussed in supervision; if necessary, there may be a change of therapist. The more serious situations, however, are those where there is either a deliberate attempt on the part of the therapist to seduce the client, or where the therapist is blind to the inappropriateness of the relationship. Here the only safeguards are the intervention of colleagues 'blowing the whistle', the use by the client of the complaints procedure, or (as in the Kerr/Haslam case) the intervention of the media and eventually the law.

One outcome of the various inquiries carried out by the Department of Health is the greater publicity that has been given to abuse of the therapist–client relationship. It is to be hoped that the generality of clients will be more aware than before of the need for therapists to respect boundaries, and to be more ready to make a complaint if there is something which seems 'not quite right' in the relationship. Deliberate transgression of boundaries will probably always occur, albeit rarely, but those which arise through excessive therapeutic enthusiasm or a misplaced belief that a sexual relationship with the client might be helpful should be reduced by increased patient awareness, better therapist training, therapist registration, more use of supervision, and a better use of colleague monitoring, whistle-blowing and the complaints procedure.

References

Crowe, M. & Ridley, J. (2000) *Therapy with Couples* (2nd edn). Blackwell.
Department of Health (2005) *The Kerr/Haslam Inquiry*. TSO (The Stationery Office).
Masters, W. H. & Johnson, V. E. (1970) *Human Sexual Inadequacy*. Little, Brown.
Tunnadine, L. P. (1970) *Contraception and Sexual Life: A Therapeutic Approach*. Tavistock.

CHAPTER 10

Obstetrics and gynaecology: a special case?

Patricia Crowley

Overview

Given that all patients in obstetrics and gynaecology are female and that the assessment of patients often involves pelvic examination, it is not surprising that sexual misconduct occurs. Measures that should reduce the incidence of misconduct include guidelines about the conduct of intimate examination, the use of chaperones, information for patients about what to expect in a gynaecology clinic and better education of doctors by their professional trainers and by nursing and midwifery colleagues. Male gynaecologists may be sometimes culturally stereotyped as sexual fantasy figures and patients may occasionally behave seductively: doctors must be trained to manage such a situation appropriately. Because of the high rates of violence against women and girls worldwide, the presence of a partner at a consultation should not be regarded as automatically beneficial. The specialty has a role in advocating women's rights to health.

Background

Doctor–patient relationships are open to abuse in all medical specialties. The specialty of obstetrics and gynaecology, however, is unique for a number of reasons: all patients are female; most obstetric patients and many seeking family planning services and cervical screening are young and healthy; a positive relationship with a midwife, general practitioner (GP) or obstetrician during these early encounters with healthcare professionals may be a valuable learning experience for a woman and may influence a family's use of healthcare services for a generation; a negative experience may have destructive consequences. Pelvic examination, either digital or by speculum, is often an essential part of the assessment of most conditions in gynaecology and may also be necessary during labour. The situation therefore exposes the patient to a very specific potential for sexual abuse.

From puberty to extreme old age, women may suffer a variety of gynaecological discomforts and minor disorders that are troublesome rather than life-threatening. This puts women at risk of excessive intervention if they encounter a gynaecologist who is eager to operate for financial or other reasons. Early exposure to respectful doctor–patient relationships with informed, shared decision-making in general practice, family planning, gynaecology or colposcopy clinics enables a woman to deal appropriately with these gynaecological disorders throughout her lifetime.

Sexual misconduct in obstetrics and gynaecology

In 2003 and 2004, the Professional Conduct Committee (PCC) of the General Medical Council (GMC) heard a total of 28 cases that involved allegations of inappropriate sexual contact with patients, which accounted for 10% of all its new disciplinary cases (Department of Health, 2005). Three-quarters of the cases resulted in a finding of serious professional misconduct. As a result, in 2004, eight doctors had their names erased from the Medical Register. Two recent cases of doctors working in obstetrics and gynaecology who were struck off for sexual misconduct are reported by way of example in Boxes 10.1 and 10.2.

Box 10.1 Clifford Ayling

In December 2000 Clifford Ayling, a general practitioner and clinical assistant in gynaecology, who had trained to registrar level in obstetrics and gynaecology, was convicted on 12 counts of indecent assault relating to 10 female patients, and sentenced to 4 years' imprisonment. The complaints of indecent assault related to inappropriate touching of breasts or gynaecological organs during the course of medical examinations.

Source: Department of Health (2004).

Box 10.2 Paul Vinall

In 2002, Paul Vinall, a consultant obstetrician gynaecologist, was given an 18-month suspended sentence after being found guilty of indecently assaulting two of his patients. He was cleared of three other charges. A further 26 charges were ordered to remain on file. Both counts involved Vinall conducting 'inappropriate' examinations on women. In both cases, the alleged incidents continued over many years of clinical practice before being detected.

Source: BBC News online, 'Gynaecologist found guilty of indecent assault, 8 March 2002, http://news.bbc.co.uk/1/hi/england/1862645.stm (accessed June 2010).

The true prevalence of sexual misconduct in the doctor–patient relationship is impossible to estimate (see Chapter 5). Lamont & Woodward's (1994) survey of 618 Canadian gynaecologists revealed that 10% admitted knowing of another colleague who had been sexually involved with a patient and 3% of male and 1% of female gynaecologists themselves admitted sexual involvement with a patient. Significantly more females reported awareness of a colleague's sexual involvement, and they supported stronger sanctions. Sexual involvement was defined by the respondents and by the College of Physicians and Surgeons of Ontario, and ranged from inviting a patient on a date, to behaviour or remarks of a sexual nature or sexual intercourse. In a questionnaire-based study in one urban and one rural general practice in Canada, 8% of women surveyed by Webb & Opdahl (1996) reported that their family doctor had been 'less than professional' (citing over-exposure of the body, inappropriate comments, gestures or facial expressions or being examined in an unusual position).

The most extreme form of sexual misconduct is for a doctor to have sexual intercourse with a patient, regardless of apparent consent. Unless unconscious or sedated, patients are well aware that this has occurred. Of great concern is the more subtle and insidious abuse constituted by inappropriate conduct of a pelvic examination, as patients may be confused about what is happening and abuse may remain undetected.

Guidelines

In 1996, the GMC issued a brief guideline on the conduct of intimate examinations. The Council of the Royal College of Obstetricians and Gynaecologists (RCOG) recognised that more specific guidelines were required for doctors practising in obstetrics and gynaecology and convened a working party, chaired by the present author. A detailed document was published in 1997 and revised in 2002, entitled *Gynaecological Examinations: Guidelines for Specialist Practice*. The key recommendations were:

- The doctor should consider what information is to be gained by the examination.
- The doctor should explain the nature and purpose of the examination and obtain verbal consent.
- Gloves should be worn on both hands.
- Patients should be provided with privacy to undress and dress. The area in which the examination takes place should be private and other individuals should not enter the room while the examination is in progress.
- Assistance with dressing or undressing should not be offered unless absolutely necessary.
- Remarks of a personal nature and terms of endearment such as 'love' and 'pet' should be avoided during pelvic examination.

- Written consent should be obtained from women undergoing procedures under anaesthesia if a medical student is to perform a pelvic examination for purposes of education or training.

Detailed consideration was also given to the patient's first vaginal examination, to the examination of women with learning disabilities and of those who had been sexually assaulted.

The original document, while welcomed by many, was regarded by some as excessively prescriptive. Experienced gynaecologists scoffed at the need to advise doctors to wear gloves on both hands. Practitioners from low-budget family planning clinics and high-profit private practices expressed dismay at the extra costs of employing paid chaperones (discussed below). However, evidence given during the Ayling and Vinall cases (Boxes 10.1 and 10.2) proved the need for such guidelines, which were cited in court during the Vinall case and referred to in the Ayling Inquiry (Department of Health, 2004). In these and other cases, complaints have been made about doctors performing pelvic examinations without gloves, watching patients undress, asking women to walk across the examination room naked, and remarking on women's physical attributes during examination. It is inappropriate to ask very personal questions while the patient is undressed or during vaginal examination.

Chaperones

The 1997 report of the RCOG Working Party on Intimate Examinations recommended that:

a chaperone should be offered to all patients undergoing intimate examination irrespective of the gender of the gynaecologist. If the patient prefers to be examined without a chaperone this request should be honoured and recorded in the notes.

The revised (2002) version states that:

the Working Party recommends that a chaperone *should be available* [emphasis added] to assist with gynaecological examinations irrespective of the gender of the gynaecologist. Ideally, this assistant should be a professional individual.

This revised version, issued after the Vinall case, was intended to strengthen the recommendation that a chaperone should be present, but it still falls short of stating that *a chaperone should be present*.

The Committee of Inquiry into Quality and Practice Within the National Health Service arising out of the actions of Rodney Ledward (whose case is discussed below – see Box 10.4) recommended (Department of Health, 2000) that all obstetric and gynaecological units should adopt the guidelines produced by the RCOG. The recommendation from the Committee of Inquiry into how the National Health Service (NHS) handled allegations in the case of Clifford Ayling is more robust than the 2002 RCOG position:

'the presence of a chaperone must be the patient's decision but must be routinely offered by a health care professional' (Department of Health, 2004: p. 26). The Committee's report also recommended that:

no family member or friend of a patient should be expected to undertake any formal chaperoning role. The presence of a chaperone during a clinical examination or treatment must be the clearly expressed choice of a patient. Chaperoning should not be undertaken by other than trained staff: the use of untrained administrative staff as chaperones in a GP's surgery, for example, is not acceptable. However, the patient must have a right to decline any chaperone offered if they so wish. (Department of Health, 2004: p. 26)

Advantages of chaperones

The presence of a chaperone acts as a safeguard both against sexual abuse by a doctor and against a doctor causing unnecessary discomfort, pain, humiliation or intimidation during examination. A chaperone may provide reassurance to an anxious patient. An experienced chaperone would identify unusual or unacceptable behaviour by a doctor during an examination and may help prevent misunderstandings and miscommunications. The presence of a chaperone may protect a doctor from a patient who behaves seductively during a clinical examination or from a patient who makes false allegations of sexual misconduct. However, it is important that this aspect of the role of chaperones is not emphasised to the detriment of the other potential benefits.

Disadvantages of chaperones

Some patients' level of embarrassment during gynaecological examination is increased in proportion to the number of individuals present. Gynaeco-logical consultations occasionally provide the opportunity for women to confide sensitive information about sexual abuse, domestic violence, a previous concealed pregnancy or termination of pregnancy and therefore the RCOG Working Party suggested that the gynaecological consultation should be one to one wherever possible, with the chaperone attending the physical examination.

Professional chaperones increase the costs of running family planning clinics or general practices. Hospital-based nurses or healthcare assistants may feel that chaperoning is an inappropriate use of their time and expertise. Lay chaperones, especially family members, may intrude in the doctor–patient relationship and may bring their own agenda of fears and prejudices about gynaecological examination to the consultations. Stern (2001), an expert in prisoners' rights, argues strongly against chaperones from a patient's perspective, believing that the patient is entitled to privacy and should be spared embarrassment and indignity. She argues that the presence of chaperones did not protect patients from physical and emotional pain at the hands of Rodney Ledward, who was struck off the register in the UK in 1998 because of malpractice (Box 10.4). However, the presence of a chaperone is normalised when the chaperone assists with adjusting the light for a speculum examination, labelling specimens and talking to the patient. Obviously, a woman who is uncomfortable with having a chaperone present has the right to refuse.

The contribution of nurses and midwives

The Royal College of Nursing (2006) has issued a comprehensive guideline on the conduct of vaginal examinations in nursing and midwifery, which deals with the role of the nurse or midwife both as the practitioner of the vaginal examination and as the chaperone. The role of the nurse or midwife as patient advocate is emphasised in this document. This is likely to improve the practice of nurses and to strengthen their effectiveness as chaperones. For instance, there is a lack of awareness among some nurses and midwives that briskly removing the underwear of a woman undergoing a vaginal examination is unnecessary and unacceptable.

Stern (2001) expressed the opinion that nurses are not equipped to supervise or control doctors. This is the personal view of an intelligent laywoman. This author disagrees. Many years in practice have left her in no doubt that midwives and experienced nurses who work in gynaecology are well equipped to detect and correct inappropriate behaviour. The report of the Committee of Inquiry into how the NHS handled allegations into the conduct of Clifford Ayling recommended that policies within NHS trusts for identifying staff concerns should specifically identify 'sexualised behaviour' by doctors during examinations as appropriate for reporting within the confidence of the 'whistle-blowing' process (Department of Health, 2004: p. 22).

Educating patients

Gawande (2007) asserts that medical examinations are 'inherently ambiguous'. Any patient can be led to wonder: Did the doctor really need to touch me there? And if so, can the ambiguity be removed, possibly by educating women about what to expect when they attend a gynaecology clinic? Women should be provided with written information before they attend colposcopy clinics and could be provided with an information leaflet regarding the normal conduct of a gynaecological clinic (see Box 10.3). A cartoon version or a DVD could be supplied for women who have poor literacy skills. A culture of greater advance knowledge of what is normal at a gynaecological examination might both reassure women and reduce the potential for inappropriate conduct of examinations.

Box 10.3 Suggested content of a patient information leaflet 'What should I expect when I attend the gynaecology clinic?'

- What should I wear?
- Should I keep my appointment if I have my period?
- What will I be asked?
- Will I have to have an internal examination?
- Who will be in the room?
- How much will I have to undress?
- Where will I undress?

Inappropriate sexual behaviour by patients

So far, appropriately, the discussion of sexualisation of the doctor–patient relationship has centred on inappropriate behaviour on the part of doctors. The doctor is in a position of power and therefore the need to avoid abuse of this power cannot be overstated. Can patients abuse the doctor–patient relationship? Most male obstetricians and gynaecologists anecdotally report experiences of patients making inappropriate sexual remarks, dressing seductively or undressing excessively when asked to prepare for examination. The internet is replete with personal accounts by women reporting that they have fallen in love with their gynaecologist. Women's magazine articles print humorous accounts of women wearing their sexiest underwear when attending a gynaecology appointment. Obstetricians and gynaecologists report no training or preparation in how to deal with the 'seductive' patient. They need to be educated in how to handle these rare situations, and need to understand that apparently 'seductive' behaviours may be a patient's way of coping with anxiety, a means of reducing the power imbalance, or even habit according to cues – which could even just be a man behaving pleasantly. Failure by the doctor to deal appropriately with these situations is indefensible and must be regarded as an abuse of the doctor–patient relationship, by the doctor.

Excessive and untried surgical intervention

In a number of high-profile cases, consultant obstetricians and gynaecologists have been struck off the Medical Registers in the UK and Ireland for excessive or negligent surgery (see Boxes 10.4 and 10.5). In most specialties, patients are heavily reliant on the advice of doctors as to the necessity of surgical intervention. There is a risk of excessive intervention where doctors are being paid on a fee-per-item basis for procedures and operations or

---

Box 10.4 Rodney Ledward – flamboyant, excessive and negligent

Rodney Ledward, a consultant gynaecologist at the William Harvey Hospital in Ashford, Kent, who dubbed himself 'the fastest gynaecologist in the south', was struck off the Medical Register in 1998 for serious professional misconduct relating to 13 operations. The Ritchie Inquiry concluded that, despite numerous complications, complaints from patients, challenges from nursing staff, management investigations, a disciplinary investigation and formal warning, it did not appear to cross his mind that there was anything amiss with his technique (Department of Health, 2000). The Inquiry uncovered evidence that he exerted pressure on women to attend him as private patients and that he pressurised them into undergoing gynaecological operations. 'A private patient told us that Rodney Ledward had carried out a laparoscopy and D&C in January 1990, a ventrosuspension in March 1990, another laparoscopy, D&C and sterilisation in October 1990, a vaginal hysterectomy in January 1991, and division of adhesions in July 1991. The patient told us that she was concerned that all these procedures might not have been necessary. We share her concern' (Department of Health, 2000: p. 37).He was flamboyant and supremely confident, sometimes turning up at a patient's bedside dressed in riding gear, wearing a buttonhole, carrying a whip or smelling of drink (Department of Health, 2000: p. 45). At least 92 women won compensation for negligence.

---

where fashions prevail. Women are vulnerable to excess intervention in both obstetric and gynaecological settings. In obstetrics, the relationship between payment method and mode of delivery has been recognised for many years. Two large studies illustrate the issue. A study of primiparous women in New York from 1996 to 2003 inclusive found a 21.2% Caesarean section rate (CSR) in 51682 women insured by Medicaid, compared with a rate of 30.4% in 321308 women who carried private health insurance (Lipkind *et al*, 2009). A population-based study from New South Wales examined intervention rates in 171157 women who delivered a live-born baby in 1996 and 1997. Private patients delivering in private hospitals had the highest intervention rates, followed by private patients in public hospitals. Publicly funded patients delivering in public hospitals had the lowest intervention rates. Notably, only 18% of privately funded primiparae in private hospitals had a vaginal birth without any intervention, compared with 29% of the private patients in public hospitals and 39% of the public patients (Roberts *et al*, 2000). The differences cannot be accounted for by differences in risk factors between the groups, which were analysed in this study. An Australian government report into childbirth procedures stated that private practice encouraged operative intervention for comparatively minor indications, not so much because doctors are paid more for Caesarean sections but because it takes longer to supervise a normal labour and delivery than to perform a Caesarean section or an instrumental vaginal delivery (Senate Community Affairs Reference Committee, 1999).

Box 10.5 Surgical saying

Good surgeons know how to operate, better surgeons when to operate and the best surgeons when not to operate.

There is a wide variation in practice between gynaecologists with respect to their threshold for recommending surgery for benign conditions such as heavy menstrual bleeding or prolapse. This may be driven by economic factors, by the gynaecologist's access to beds and theatre time, and by how much the gynaecologist enjoys operating, none of which is an appropriate reason for varying standards. The commonest benign gynaecological condition is excessive menstrual blood loss, with a third of all menstruating women reporting heavy periods (Kennedy *et al*, 2002). In the 1990s, it was estimated that 20% of women in the UK would undergo hysterectomy by age 55 (Vessey *et al*, 1992). Since then, new interventions such as endometrial ablation and the levonorgestrel intrauterine system have become available for the treatment of excessive menstrual blood loss. A randomised controlled trial of providing a structured interview to assist women with making decisions about management of heavy menstrual bleeding showed a substantial reduction in the rates of hysterectomy in those randomised to the structured interview (Kennedy *et al*, 2002).

The development of laparoscopic and robotic techniques for gynaeco-logical surgery opens up the possibility of new forms of abuse of the doctor–patient relationship. Laparoscopic hysterectomy, total laparoscopic hysterectomy and robotic hysterectomy are seductive new techniques being driven forward by enthusiasts and backed by commercial interests. Although a series of over 3000 laparoscopic hysterectomies for benign disease performed by a single team (Donnez *et al*, 2009) had an impressively low complication rate, a Cochrane review (Johnson *et al*, 2009) of 34 randomised trials showed that vaginal hysterectomy was associated with the best outcomes. Laparoscopic hysterectomies were associated with an increased incidence of bladder and ureteric injuries.

Clearly, it is appropriate to innovate and develop surgical techniques that may reduce hospital stay and shorten the return to normal activities. Women are vulnerable to persuasion, as they will be quick to consent to procedures that are cosmetically acceptable, avoid large incisions and offer a shorter hospital stay. They must be informed of the risk of complications and need to know how the gynaecologist who is proposing to perform the surgery is progressing on the steep learning curve associated with new surgical interventions. Abenhaim *et al* (2008) analysed 341 487 hysterectomies performed in the USA between 1998 and 2002. They showed that the major determinant of whether a woman underwent abdominal hysterectomy or laparoscopic hysterectomy was median household income. Women with private insurance were more likely to undergo hysterectomy laparoscopically. The wealthier they were, the more likely this was to happen. The authors interpret these results as evidence of unequal access to care. However, it may be that, in this case, poorer women were being spared unnecessary complications incurred while gynaecologists honed their new surgical techniques. A recent call for an improved code of practice in the evaluation of new surgical techniques may eventually protect both women and men from excessive enthusiasm for new techniques (McCulloch *et al*, 2009).

Pressure from patients to intervene

All obstetricians and gynaecologists have encountered cases where patients have demanded unnecessary interventions. Doctors can feel professionally disempowered if they are forced to perform what they believe to be an unnecessary operation (whether on the demand of the patient, or during training, on the instruction of a senior, with whom they disagree). Obstetricians and gynaecologists need increased training in how to deal with these requests, in particular how to explore the reasons why a woman is intent on a particular intervention, such as a Caesarean section or a hysterectomy, for no apparent reason. They may find it hard to say 'no', but that is what the ethics of 'first of all, do no harm' may demand. Obstetricians and gynaecologists have been characterised as particularly paternalistic in the past, but that is no excuse for lazy or simplistic responses to complex consultations (Box 10.6). A second opinion from a colleague with a high threshold for surgical intervention may be helpful. An evaluation by a clinical psychologist may uncover the background to a request for surgery.

In vitro fertilisation (IVF) is an area where women may press for excessive intervention (Box 10.6). Their judgement may be clouded by the emotional trauma of sub-fertility and by the economic burden of paying for IVF. Intense pressure from women to implant an unsafe number of embryos, or to persist with an IVF cycle where ovarian hyperstimulation syndrome is anticipated, is a distortion of and threat to the doctor–patient relationship. Once again, a doctor who succumbs to such pressure and acts against the woman's best interests is abusing the doctor–patient relationship.

Can excessive intervention be prevented?

Audit at local or national level or through health insurers may detect statistical outliers – gynaecologists who over-operate. In the UK, regulation of the fertility sector by the Human Fertilisation and Embryology Authority ensures that a maximum of two embryos (except in women over 40) are transferred. An expert group recommended that single-embryo transfer should become the norm in the UK, as it is in publicly funded IVF in Sweden

---

Box 10.6 Excessive IVF and embryo transfer

In January 2009, a Californian, Nadya Suleman, gave birth to octuplets conceived following IVF conducted by Dr Michael Kamrava. Nadya Suleman had
six embryos remaining from previous IVF treatments transferred, despite being
informed that the recommended guideline limit was three for a woman her age
(two in the UK). She claimed part of her reasoning for attempting another pregnancy was so that the remaining embryos would not be destroyed. Six embryos
were transferred, of which two developed into identical twins, resulting in eight
babies. Dr Kamrava was expelled from the American Society for Reproductive
Medicine in October 2009.

Source: *Daily Telegraph*, 19 October 2009, 'Octomoms Dr Michael Kamrava expelled
from American Society for Reproductive Medicine', online at http://www.telegraph.co.uk/
news/newstopics/celebritynews/6380099/Octomoms-Dr-Michael-Kamrava-expelled-from-
American-Society-for-Reproductive-Medicine.html (accessed June 2010).

(Le Page, 2006). Public funding of fertility interventions may reduce the
pressure on patients to wish for more embryos to be transferred to increase
the chance of success, because each attempt costs so much.

The presence of a third party

The past three decades have seen increasing involvement of partners or
other relatives in antenatal care and labour. Although protected one-to-one
consultation time is recommended, it is now possible for a woman to go
through an entire pregnancy and delivery without a confidential consultation
with a midwife, general practitioner or obstetrician. All the evidence is
that this huge social change is what most women want. However, there
are potential disadvantages to the quality of history taking (e.g. relevant
information about sexually transmitted infections, abortions, adoption). A
significant proportion of women worldwide experience domestic violence
during pregnancy, with serious and potentially fatal consequences (Cook
& Bewley, 2008), and abusive partners are likely to control women's
reproductive choices.

The inability of women to experience antenatal consultations without the
presence of third parties reduces opportunities for the detection of domestic
violence and increases the opportunity for partners to control women's
reproductive decisions. Many obstetric units now encourage women to
carry their own case notes and most women who have participated in trials
of this policy would like to follow the same practice in a future pregnancy
(Brown & Smith, 2007). However, this practice further increases the power
of controlling partners, who may take ownership of a woman's confidential
medical history.

The constant presence of a partner or other family member during consultations reduces the possibility of a woman developing skills in articulating her fears and wishes and becoming experienced in negotiating her own healthcare decisions. As the presence of third parties at obstetric consultations becomes the norm, partners or other third parties may see attendance at gynaecological consultations as a right. It is high time for obstetricians and gynaecologists to reaffirm the confidentiality of the doctor–patient consultation and to create a climate of trust and mutual respect, where women are facilitated in developing autonomy, provided with good-quality evidence and encouraged to make decisions about their care.

Conclusion

The potential for women to be abused by obstetricians, gynaecologists and general practitioners during the course of pelvic examinations and in reaching decisions about surgical procedures arises from the imbalance of power between doctors and patients. This potential for abuse has deep-seated cultural and political roots.

There are some inherent tensions in the attributes required of obstetricians and gynaecologists: good communication skills are prized by colleagues and patients, but patients must be protected from the charming 'salesmen' who may persuade women to undergo unnecessary intervention or who 'sexualise' the consultation. Innovators and enthusiasts are essential in every branch of medicine and such individuals have in the past saved lives and improved the quality of lives; can innovators question and doubt the value of their own innovations and be persuaded to submit them to rigorous research? Obstetricians and gynaecologists should practise according to professional guidelines, but also should have the independence to recognise that some women's needs will be served by departing from the guidelines. In order to manage emergencies such as massive haemorrhage, obstetricians are required to have both teamwork and leadership skills, self-confidence, decisiveness and determination to the point of stubbornness. The challenge for the profession is to select and train candidates with these skills, while fostering the individual and institutional self-criticism required to ensure women are not betrayed by arrogant and opinionated doctors. The increasing feminisation of the workforce, however, should not lead to a sense of complacency, as women may be capable of repeating some, or all, of the offences of the past.

References

Abenhaim, H. A., Azziz, R., Hu, J., *et al* (2008) Socioeconomic and racial predictors of undergoing laparoscopic hysterectomy for selected benign disease: analysis of 341,487 hysterectomies. *Journal of Minimally Invasive Gynecology*, **15**, 11–15.

Brown, H. C. & Smith, H. J. (2007) Giving women their own case notes to carry during pregnancy. *Cochrane Database of Systematic Reviews*, **(2)**, CD002856.

Cook, J. & Bewley, S. (2008) Acknowledging a persistent truth: domestic violence in pregnancy. *Journal of the Royal Society of Medicine*, **101**, 358–363.

Department of Health (2000) *The Report of the Inquiry into the Quality and Practice Within the National Health Service Arising from the Actions of Rodney Ledward*. TSO (The Stationery Office).

Department of Health (2004) *Committee of Inquiry – Independent Investigation into How the NHS Handled Allegations into the Conduct of Clifford Ayling*. Department of Health. Available online at http://www.dh.gov.uk/en/Publicationsandstatistics/Publications/PublicationsPolicyAndGuidance/DH_4088996 (accessed June 2010).

Department of Health (2005) *The Kerr/Haslam Inquiry*. TSO (The Stationery Office).

Donnez, O., Jadoul, P., Squifflet, J., *et al* (2009) A series of 3190 laparoscopic hysterectomies for benign disease from 1990 to 2006: evaluation of complications compared with vaginal and abdominal procedures. *British Journal of Obstetrics and Gynaecology*, **116**, 492–500.

Gawande, A. (2007) Naked. In *Better. A Surgeon's Notes on Performance*, pp 73–83. Picador.

General Medical Council (1996) *Intimate Examinations*. GMC.

Johnson, N., Barlow, D., Lethaby, A., *et al* (2009) Surgical approach to hysterectomy for benign disease. *Cochrane Database of Systematic Reviews*, **(3)**, CD003677.

Kennedy, A. D., Sculpher, M. J., Coulter, A., *et al* (2002) Effects of decision aids for menorrhagia on treatment choices, health outcomes and costs. *JAMA*, **288**, 2701–2708.

Lamont, J. A. & Woodward, C. (1994) Patient–physician sexual involvement: a Canadian survey of obstetrician-gynaecologists. *Canadian Medical Association Journal*, **150**, 1433–1439.

Le Page, M. (2006) Fertility experts call for one embryo per IVF cycle. Available online at http://www.newscientist.com/article/dn10326-fertility-experts-call-for-one-embryo-per-ivf-cycle.html.

Lipkind, H. S., Duzyi, C., Rosenberg, T. J., *et al* (2009) Disparities in Caesarean delivery rates and associated adverse neonatal outcomes in New York City hospitals. *Obstetrics and Gynecology*, **113**, 1239–1247.

McCulloch, P., Altman, D., Bruce Campbell, W., *et al* (2009) No surgical innovation without evaluation: the IDEAL recommendation. *Lancet*, **374**, 1105–1112.

Roberts, C. L., Tracy, S. & Peal, B. (2000) Rates for obstetric intervention among private and public patients in Australia: population based descriptive study. *BMJ*, **321**, 137–141.

Royal College of Nursing (2006) *Vaginal and Pelvic Examination. Guidelines for Nurses and Midwives*. Royal College of Nursing.

Royal College of Obstetricians and Gynaecologists (1997) *Intimate Examinations. Report of a Working Party*. RCOG Press.

Royal College of Obstetricians and Gynaecologists (2002) *Gynaecological Examinations: Guidelines for Specialist Practice*. RCOG Press.

Senate Community Affairs Reference Committee (1999) *Rocking the Cradle: A Report of Childbirth Procedures*. Commonwealth of Australia.

Stern, V. (2001) Gynaecological examination post-Ledward – a private matter. *Lancet*, **358**, 1896–1898.

Vessey, M. P., Villard-Mackintosh, L., McPherson, K., *et al* (1992) The epidemiology of hysterectomy: findings of a large cohort study. *British Journal of Obstetrics and Gynaecology*, **99**, 402–407.

Webb, R. & Opdahl, M. (1996) Breast and pelvic examinations: easing women's discomfort. *Canadian Family Physician*, **42**, 54–58.

CHAPTER 11

Nurses as abusers: a career perspective

Peter Carter

Overview

Abuses of the carer–patient relationship occur outside medicine and psycho-therapy. Nurses have day-to-day contact with in-patients and those in community care, and also have the potential to abuse patients, though not necessarily sexually. This chapter explores the stresses and problems that lead nurses to fall from the highest standards of patient care. Those nurses who do abuse patients may be suffering more from burnout, demoralisation and distress than those who maintain an ethical approach. The chapter includes examples of nurses who speak of their abuse of patients, and attempts to explain the origins of the abuse in these cases. An example is given of good practice in response to a complaint against a nurse who was found by an industrial tribunal to have physically abused a patient with psychosis, although the patient was at first not believed.

Introduction

As a student nurse in 1970, I witnessed a male nurse administering an enema in a cruel and forceful manner to a frail elderly man who had been in a mental hospital for most of his adult life. This man, bereft of any friends and family, suffered a wretched existence in an overcrowded and under-resourced ward with a maximum of three nursing staff on duty at any one time for 44 patients. I asked why the nurse had to be so rough. Was there not an alternative to assisting the patient to open his bowels other than via an enema? It was explained that the patient frequently suffered from constipation and that an enema was the only effective way of 'dealing with him'. The patient disliked the tube being inserted into him. However, as he was so frail, any attempt to prevent it could hardly be described as 'resistant to treatment', which is the expression the male nurse used. It occurred to me that the patient's reluctance had more to do with the attitude of the nurse than a conscious decision to resist the enema. In attempting to justify his conduct the nurse stated that in nursing you sometimes have to be 'cruel to be kind'.

In a sympathetic discussion with an experienced colleague it was clear that within the old mental hospital system there was a tolerance of mistreatment of patients. Many reasons were put forward to explain poor practice, such as low staffing, isolation, low expectations from relatives, and a low expectation from staff of their ability to help.

Why do nurses abuse patients?

At the annual conference of the Psychiatric Nurses Association in 1981, in response to a talk on allegations of mistreatment, a delegate and manager of a community nursing service, Tom McKervey, asked why there was so little research into understanding why nursing staff might abuse patients. He made the point that, in his experience, when an allegation of mistreatment occurred, everything was geared to the investigation. This would ultimately decide whether or not the allegation was proven. If so, appropriate action would be taken against the nurse. 'People do not come into nursing to abuse people, so why do some end up doing it? Do we not owe a responsibility to our staff, ourselves and our patients to try to examine the reasons why abuse might occur?' (cited in Carter, 1998, p. 2).

In a career spanning over 30 years in the National Health Service (NHS) I have had the privilege of working with innumerable dedicated and conscientious people. These individuals were often working in unglamorous clinical settings, such as long-stay wards in mental handicap and mental illness hospitals, geriatric and psycho-geriatric wards, or in settings where people are suffering from long-standing physical illnesses such as brain injuries or chronic conditions such as multiple sclerosis. It is therefore important to state that the vast majority of staff with whom I have worked in the NHS appear to have all the right qualities required to work with the sick and the vulnerable.

However, throughout this time I have also been aware that in many hospitals and institutions there are some staff whose conduct is completely alien to the culture and concept of nursing – that is, always to help and assist those in need of care. There has been a lack of awareness and attention to the issue of patient abuse in the nursing profession. When a scandal has broken in the public arena, much reliance has been placed by senior nursing staff on statements such as 'there is always one rotten apple in the barrel' or that the odd person 'cracks under stress'. This is too simplistic. There must be a whole range of reasons why nursing staff might abuse patients. The analogies simply fail to explain why a person might be inappropriately recruited to nursing or why an 'apple' (person) might turn rotten. The profession also fails in its responsibility to understand why some nursing staff might 'crack'. Which nurses crack? Are there any common factors? Why do NHS trusts, hospitals, health authorities not collect and routinely monitor allegations and the incidence of abuse? When there is a specific incident in a hospital there may be an internal investigation or external inquiry, but it is rare that issues are examined in a longitudinal context, or routinely monitored.

I believe that working in the nursing profession requires the skills of tolerance, perseverance and sensitivity. These skills are hard to identify in the artificial setting of conventional recruitment interviews and may be truly identified and honed only when a person has been exposed to the rigours of nursing. There is an inherent failure to monitor and support nursing staff in a meaningful way throughout their career. Thus, if a nurse starts to behave in a hitherto alien way, there are few systems and processes within the NHS to identify and intervene constructively.

Despite years of concern over the many scandals and the subsequent inquiries concerning the conduct of nursing staff in the treatment of people with mental illness or intellectual disability, there is surprisingly little research into the subject. What has been written seems to be largely qualitative and descriptive.

Types of abuse and the context

Jim Marr, the chair of a Royal College of Nursing (RCN) Special Interest Group in Elderly Care (reported by Miller, 1996), looked at the hidden abuse of elderly people in institutional care and identified four categories:

- infantilisation – treating people as irresponsible children, for example subjecting them to toileting regimes and scolding them for bad table manners
- depersonalisation – when services such as bathing, feeding and toileting are provided on an assembly-line basis
- dehumanisation – where the older person is ignored as a person, has no privacy, and lacks power, choice and respect
- victimisation – when the older person's physical and moral integrity is attacked through theft, blackmail, punishment and rough handling.

Marr added that some of these situations were brought about by staff demoralisation, the creation of authoritarian cultures, emotional exhaustion, ignorance, the failure of audit and unthinking care regimens.

The well-respected publication *Hospitals in Trouble* (Martin, 1984) has been recommended as standard reading for each new generation of student nurses. Martin charted the problems that were experienced in Britain's mental hospitals from the mid-1960s with the publication of the 'Sans Everything' letter in November 1965: through the troubled years of hospital inquiries, the emergence of the Hospital Advisory Service, the publication of numerous reports on how to improve services, into the early 1980s, when the fashion for major national inquiries into poor practice changed and emphasis was placed on local health authorities' responsibility to address matters of concern. The chapter 'Helping staff' (Martin, 1984, pp. 218–240) attempted to elucidate the pressures and difficulties staff face in coping in circumstances and with resources that are often less than adequate or desirable and are not conducive to a positive working life. Martin set out three factors that may help to understand why some staff at times behave inappropriately to the patients they are charged with caring for:

- The fundamental problem with working with people who are chronically ill, the elderly or those with severe handicaps, most of whom will be in care for long periods, may be the lack of achievement. Caring for the acutely ill may have its failures but this is usually offset by success and thus staff morale can be boosted by positive results.
- The emphasis in mental illness, as in physical illness, on the acutely ill patient has usually meant that staffing ratios are poorer for the more dependent patients. Consequently, all are working closer to the lowest acceptable standards of care. Hence merely coping with the strains of work to achieve a degree of order among more disturbed patients makes heavy demands on physical and, especially, mental stamina.
- Those working with long-stay patients can become professionally isolated and fail to realise when their methods become outdated. Isolation easily breeds stagnation. 'Our methods' become '*the* methods'. Pressure of work can reinforce the old task-centred nursing with its underlying assumptions of the unimportance of the individual in relation to the organisation's routines. Martin makes reference (p. 219) to the work of Audrey John, who, in *A Study of the Psychiatric Nurse* (1961), stresses the extent to which conformity with routines was regarded as the mark of a 'good' patient.

The work of Martin is as relevant today as when it was first published. It is depressing that many of the indicators set out by Martin in relation to abuse and neglect have still not been adopted.

The abuse of patients is often associated with remote, isolated institutions, with people who have severe and enduring mental health problems, or an intellectual difficulty, and who often lack the capacity to raise issues and complaints. However, these factors were certainly not present in the case of Britten (see Box 11.1). The events which surrounded that case, which were brought to light only recently, are a pertinent reminder that abuse can take place in high-profile environments that are regularly visited, inspected, regulated and can be regarded as exemplary. The case also reveals the difficulties with prosecuting such abusers.

Nursing – a stressful occupation

Concern over the stress factors in nursing goes back many years. Research has consistently shown that nursing is an occupation that at times

Box 11.1 David Britten

Over a period of 20 years within the Peter Dally Eating Disorder Clinic in central London, David Britten systematically sexually abused young women who were suffering from eating disorders. In many cases this involved cuddling, kissing and full sex. An independent inquiry (McKenna & Hussain, 2008) demonstrated that he had managed to build up a regimen wherein he acted with impunity. The women at the unit were emotionally and psychologically dependent upon him, and were compliant with his demands. Over the years, there were occasions when Britten's victims raised concerns and sought help from other professionals, carers and relatives. However, the response, especially from professionals, was frequently to 'pathologise' the patients' complaints and to interpret the allegations that Britten was behaving inappropriately as a manifestation of illness. The women were frequently seen as attention seeking and manipulative, exhibiting aberrant behaviours associated with borderline personality disorder and eating disorder. I believe that, as a result of this, Britten was able to 'trade off' their illnesses, and thus conduct himself with confidence that his behaviour would not be exposed. This took place in a high-profile unit in which student nurses, junior doctors and other professionals trained over many years: the unit itself was frequently held up by the Riverside Mental Health Trust that managed it as a model of good practice.

Britten was very careful that all of his victims were over the age of 16 and none of them was on a detention order of the Mental Health Act at the time the abuse took place. All of his victims acknowledged they were compliant at the time. Consequently, although Britten was dismissed and struck off the Nursing Register, the Crown Prosecution Service believed that it would be unable to secure a conviction. Britten is now thought to be living in the Philippines.

demonstrates characteristics that give significant cause for concern. Hingley & Cooper (1986) suggested that nurses are a high-risk group in relation to alcohol misuse and that nurses appear to suffer abnormally high suicide rates. Booth (1985) drew attention to the fact that a growing number of nursing staff were presenting themselves to treatment centres for help with their drinking problems. Information from the Office of Population Censuses and Surveys (1978) on the mortality of female workers suggested that women nurses were more likely to commit suicide than women in any other profession. Hingley & Cooper's (1986) research demonstrates that while smoking at that time among nurses was no higher than among women in general (25%), the rate remained static, unlike the national trend, which showed a rapidly decreasing level of consumption. Carson *et al* (1995) examined the relationship among mental health nurses between self-esteem and stress, coping and burnout. One of the key moderating variables in determining the effects of stress on individuals is self-esteem. In conducting their study, Carson *et al* found that nurses who had low self-esteem were more likely to smoke and to drink frequently. They further identified that nurses who had low job satisfaction had low self-esteem. These nurses were also:

- more psychologically distressed
- more emotionally exhausted
- more depersonalised
- more burned out
- less personally accomplished
- twice as likely to take sick leave.

The study also revealed that factors associated with high self-esteem included:

- good physical fitness
- job security
- having a supportive relationship with the line manager
- having children.

A number of other articles over recent years have examined these issues further.

Davis (2000) discusses occupational stress levels and depression among nurses. Using figures published by the Office for National Statistics, Meitzer *et al* (2008) point out that those working as health professionals had among the highest suicide rates, and highlight the fact that nurses in particular have significantly high suicide rates. The possibility of a link between increasing workloads and alcohol use by nurses is suggested by Cooper (2000) from the results of an alcohol use questionnaire.

Irving (2004) analysed the reasons why stress levels and suicide rates among NHS staff are high. Particular concerns included experiences of harassment, bullying or abuse, work patterns, fatigue and poor working environments. O'Dowd (2006) examined the incidence of alcohol misuse among nurses and the failure of many nurses to seek help if they have an alcohol-related problem. The effects of occupational stress on nurses' health and well-being were researched by a survey on nurses' experiences of stress by the *Nursing Times* (Vere-Jones, 2007). The work-related reasons for stress and the impact on nurses' sickness absence, alcohol consumption, smoking and sexual and emotional relationships are discussed.

Nurses who have abused patients speak

The series of anonymised vignettes presented in Boxes 11.2–11.5 come from interviews with nurses who have abused patients (and who gave permission for their use). This is a limited sample, as it is hard to find nurses who are prepared to talk openly. Although these relate to specific cases, they nevertheless give interesting insights into the types of circumstances in which nurses were accused of abusing patients, how they reacted and the reaction of their employers.

Box 11.2 Charge nurse hits an elderly patient

A charge nurse in psychiatric nursing, who had qualified 25 years previously, was found guilty of hitting an elderly patient and dismissed. The nurse commented:

'I lost my way. I had been in this particular role for 10 years. I did not have any real insight into my conduct until a student nurse reported me. Basically I was struggling to get a difficult patient undressed for bed, and he was being resistive. He scratched and spat at me. I punched him in the stomach – not particularly hard – but it had the desired effect of making him cooperate. There is a lot I could say. Overall I wished I'd moved on and not allowed myself to be stuck in a rut. I accept that I have the responsibility for this, but I also think that managers should have helped me. For years I worked in a stressful environment with low staffing levels. I know that after I left staffing was increased. It certainly suited the management to leave me in an understaffed ward where I was viewed as someone who could cope.'

Box 11.3 Ward sister with a poor attitude to patients

A ward sister had worked on a ward for elderly patients for 31 years at the time of the accusation and for 21 years as a ward sister at the hospital. She was accused by a nursing auxiliary of having a very poor attitude to patients and was cited as being intolerant and rigid in her approach, at times either scolding patients as if they were disobedient children, or publicly berating them for their 'behavioural problems' such as incontinence. She stated:

'At the time the nursing auxiliary reported me, I was very upset and angry. But as the allegations unfolded, and particularly when I saw them set out in writing, and read the nursing auxiliary's statement, I reluctantly began to look at myself. It was also during this time that I had problems with my home life and my husband and myself were separating after 20 years of marriage. I was given good advice and support by a senior manager and at the hearing I acknowledged that some of the things attributed to me were true, although I did make the point that the nursing auxiliary was a very sensitive individual. I also made the point that I had a good record and that I had always been praised for running a good ward. Many relatives spoke in favour of me and I was given a final written warning and transferred to another ward. I feel the punishment was harsh and I think my immediate manager should have been criticised, as he regularly came to my ward and I never changed the way in which I conducted myself in front of him. My career is back online, and although I am soon to retire, I feel like I have given good care in my nursing, although I accept that I had been behaving in a way that was not appropriate.'

Box. 11.4 Charge nurse accused of having a sexual relationship with a patient

A charge nurse in a psychiatric unit with 18 years' experience, who had been in his current role for 10 years, was accused by a former in-patient of having a sexual relationship with her and was dismissed. He said:

'I believe I was a good nurse with good prospects. I was RMN and RGN and worked in a busy acute psychiatric unit. I had marital problems and was separated from my wife. I admit that I fell for a patient, she was attractive and we got on very well. After she was discharged from the unit we met for a drink on a number of occasions. She was at that time a day patient and regularly came to the day hospital attached to the acute admission unit. After a while we began to have sexual intercourse. Of course I know that I shouldn't have done it and I knew at the time that I was putting my job and my career at risk. I really don't think there's too much else I can say about it. I knew what I was doing. The galling thing is that I really did feel very attracted to the woman, who also happened to be a patient. Although the relationship didn't last, in the early stages we both seemed to get a great deal from it. I think I should add that it was only when I finished the relationship that the patient reported me; she said that she felt I'd taken advantage of her. I don't think this is strictly true: she was fully compliant and there was no way that I forced her. I think it was only in retrospect, after it had finished, probably encouraged by her friends, that she reported me. I am no longer in nursing, I am no longer registered, and although I have a number of regrets I don't think my talents are best used working as a driver and I consider that the episode is closed.'

Box. 11.5 A ward sister accused of hitting a patient

A ward sister was accused by a group of staff of hitting a patient. She was dismissed from the job and has long since retired. She stated:

'My standards really slipped. I had been in nursing for 27 years and in the same job for 20 years and found it hard to accept and adapt to new ideas that were coming from student nurses and other nurses who were much more junior to me. It wasn't until the problems reached a head that friends told me that I'd become just like one of those ward sisters that I used to complain about in my youth. Unfortunately, my intolerance was not confined to the staff and I did strike a female patient who wouldn't do as I asked her. I felt it was more a push than hitting, though a number of those who gave evidence against me said I'd hit her. When I started off in nursing I saw many worse things in the hospital I trained in than I was involved in, and years ago my incident would not have been rated as an issue.'

A good practice case

There have been many complaints by patients of rough or abusive treatment by nurses. Box 11.6 presents a fictionalised account of such a complaint,

Box 11.6 Good practice in response to a complaint

A 50-year-old woman with a psychosis was a long-term patient who had spent many years in in-patient care. She could be articulate, but also had been in the habit of making complaints about members of staff in what seemed a capricious way. On this occasion she complained that a female nurse had dragged her across a room, causing abrasions on her back. The abrasions were seen by another staff member, who reported the incident to a senior manager.

The nurse was someone who had never been complained about before, but in spite of this the manager felt that the incident was serious enough to be investigated fully.

No other staff members were present when the incident occurred, but another (male) patient had observed the incident and corroborated the patient's account. This witness was more disturbed than the patient who had complained, was constantly hallucinating but gave a coherent account. The alleged perpetrator denied the incident, and contended that the patient had injured herself deliberately by sliding down a flight of stairs.

The manager had a difficult series of decisions to make, because the nurse was well respected and so far blame-free in her career, and the two patients were not seen as good witnesses. He sought the opinion of a consultant psychiatrist, who agreed that both patients had adequate testamentary capacity despite their chronic illnesses, and could be relied upon to give evidence for the purpose of the investigation. On the other hand, it was decided by the police, who had also been informed, that a criminal prosecution could not be brought as there was no chance of proving the offence 'beyond reasonable doubt'.

At the disciplinary hearing the nurse's colleagues all supported her, and confirmed that the patient had a history of making unsubstantiated complaints. The psychiatrist, however, felt that both patients were probably telling the truth, were unlikely to have conspired to damage the nurse, and stated 'I only wish I did not believe that they were telling me the truth'. The nurse was summarily dismissed for misconduct.

At the subsequent appeal the injured patient became so disturbed that she was unable to speak. However, the other patient, while still hallucinating, gave a consistent account of the incident. The dismissal of the nurse was upheld and the investigation was judged to have been fair.

An industrial tribunal for unfair dismissal was then held, at which the nurse maintained that both the patient who had complained and the other patient were long-standing psychiatric patients and therefore unreliable witnesses. The manager, however, made the case that managers have a responsibility to ensure that patients who suffer from mental illness should be taken seriously when they make complaints as well as a duty to protect staff from spurious, illogical or malicious allegations. The need to address the concerns of patients with mental health problems was felt to be inadequately dealt with in the sub-culture of many such units. In this case the need to take patients seriously outweighed the need to protect staff. The tribunal unanimously upheld the manager's decision to dismiss the nurse, and was complimentary about the way in which the safeguards required to protect both mental health workers and the patients in their care had been addressed in the original investigation.

with details incorporated from several different cases. It sets out a real dilemma facing managers. Working with people with mental health problems can be very demanding, but abuse of patients clearly cannot be tolerated. Any action taken against staff must be properly thought through. In many situations, the patient's initial complaint would not have been taken seriously. Managers would have felt unable to act because of what could be seen as the intrinsic unreliability of people with a severe and enduring mental health problem. In this case the psychiatrist's report was critical to the investigation.

The time and effort required to follow such cases to a conclusion are immense and the burden placed on the managers is significant. Nevertheless, such cases set a tone and a culture throughout the organisation which demonstrates that users of the service (patients) are taken seriously. The senior manager here showed qualities of integrity, persistence and stamina, and made good use of clinical and managerial experience. In the absence of managers with these qualities, or the will of an organisation to follow things through despite the cost, it is not surprising that similar matters frequently are not pursued. A key point commented upon by the tribunal in its judgement was that the fact that someone has a severe and enduring mental health problem does not mean that he or she is a liar or is fundamentally unreliable. The events also clarified to staff that they were working in an organisation where abuse of patients would not go unchecked.

Conclusion

Abuse is much more prevalent in the health service than is commonly believed and should be discussed far more openly. This lack of awareness starts at the most senior echelons and works through to the clinical area. It may result in poor nurses and other practitioners being allowed to continue to practise for many years. Their abusive behaviour may never be exposed or addressed. NHS managers should be educated on how to monitor services in relation to abuse and how to investigate matters when accusations have been made.

Nursing is a profession with high stress levels, which take their toll on nurses' professionalism, as evidenced by the high suicide rate, high levels of sick leave and high referrals to clinics for alcohol misuse. More work should be undertaken to investigate the relevant stress factors and more comprehensive support mechanisms should be available. The stresses are not adequately recognised by senior managers and there is something in the culture of nursing which prevents individuals from being able to come forward and declare that they are feeling under stress or pressure. Many nurses may practise with little or no monitoring while suffering from alcoholism or an array of stress-related disorders known by others but not referred to people in authority who may be able to assist. Meanwhile, in the clinical area there is a misguided sense of loyalty among nursing staff regarding to how to react and support staff when things appear to be going wrong. Allegations of abuse and mistreatment are usually brought into the open by 'marginal' people, such as student nurses, students working on holiday placements at hospitals, visitors, relatives or users of the service themselves.

Professionals of all disciplines, especially in mental health, should avoid 'pathologising' patients and service users when concerns or complaints are raised, as this can be the vulnerability that the most exploitative abusers use to cover their crimes.

References

Booth, P. (1985) Back on the rails. Helpful nurses who bring their alcohol or drink problems to work. *Nursing Times*, **81**(35), 16–17.

Carson, J., Fagin, L. & Writter, S. (1995) *Stress and Coping in Mental Health Nursing*. Chapman & Hall.

Carter, P. J. (1998) *Understanding Reasons Why Nursing Staff and Care Workers Abuse Patients and Clients in Their Care*. PhD Thesis, University of Birmingham.

Cooper, D. (2000) Is work driving you to drink? *Nursing Times*, **96**(24), 28–31.

Davis, C. (2000) How to survive in one piece. *Nursing Times*, **96**(48), 29.

Hingley, P. & Cooper, C. (1986) *Stress and the Nurse Manager*. Wiley.

Irving, S. (2004) At breaking point. *Public Health News*, 19 July.

John, A. (1961) *A Study of the Psychiatric Nurse*. Livingstone.

Martin, J. P. (1984) *Hospitals in Trouble*. Basil Blackwell.

McKenna, A. & Hussain, T. (2008) *An Independent Investigation into the Conduct of David Britten at the Peter Dally Clinic*. Verita.

Meitzer, H., Griffiths, C., Brock, A., *et al* (2008) Patterns of suicide by occupation in England and Wales: 2001–2005. *British Journal of Psychiatry*, **193**, 73–76.

Miller, B. (1996) The final betrayal. *Health Service Journal*, **106**, 14–15.

O'Dowd, A. (2006) Drink problem. *Nursing Times*, **102**(34), 18–19.

Office of Population Censuses and Surveys (1978) *Occupational Mortality: The Registrar General's Decennial Supplement for England & Wales 1970–72*. HMSO.

Vere-Jones, E. (2007) Harming the healers. *Nursing Times*, **103**(27), 16–17.

CHAPTER 12

Medical management: governance and sexual boundary issues

Fiona Subotsky

Overview

While boundary violations occur at the level of the clinician and patient, much less attention has been paid to what could be done at an organisational level. It is well known that abuse of various kinds, sometimes systematic, can occur within institutions. This is particularly relevant in the UK, where most health encounters occur within the National Health Service and individual 'office practice' is comparatively rare. Groups of hospitals, community clinics and teams are frequently managed within trusts, which also work with voluntary and private providers, as well as social services. All have their own governance needs to ensure a high quality of patient care, and should recognise the issue of potential abuse of patients by staff. Policies alone can support change, though not ensure it, but it is undoubtedly time to lower patient risk. This chapter is aimed particularly at medical managers and makes a number of recommendations for organisations, covering principles, policies, clinical practice, staff and patient issues, and how to make best use of existing systems to achieve safer practice.

Principles

Trusts are responsible for their patients' and staff's welfare and safety, and cannot assume that everyone knows or is committed to the idea that sexual or other harassment of patients or staff is unacceptable. The first step therefore is to make this clear. The importance of being proactive, apart from the intrinsic morality and duty to prevent harm, is that sexual harassment of a variety of kinds is common, and can go on for years without being acted against. It is not enough to rely upon 'professional codes' and their regulatory enforcement, although these may help. Recent guidance from the General Medical Council (GMC) on this topic – *Maintaining Boundaries* (2006) – is strongly recommended, as are the recommendations of the Council for Healthcare Regulatory Excellence (2008).

Sexual harassment and abuse of patients by doctors can fall into any, or all, of the following categories of transgression:

- against trust disciplinary codes and policies
- against guidelines produced by the relevant Royal College
- against GMC guidelines
- against the law.

All have their own methods of investigation and sanctions, which unfortunately may be at cross-purposes with each other, and so clear liaison links and responsibility are vital. While College and GMC guidelines have been revised, and the legal situation changed with the Sexual Offences Act 2003 (Home Office, 2004), the employer has a primary responsibility for setting clear standards and ensuring enforcement. Trust policies should apply to all staff, not just clinicians, and be explicit about what sorts of behaviour are acceptable and which are not acceptable. They should include what sorts of 'touch' are allowable, whether exceptions about sexual relationships are permissible with 'former patients' and, if so, how this could be defined. If there has been a pre-existing, or there is a current, such relationship with a patient or carer, it should be the responsibility of the member of staff to discuss this with a manager. Other boundary issues, such as socialising or financial transactions, also need discussion, as they can be part of a 'slippery slope'. In addition, supportive 'whistle-blowing' policies are essential so that staff, regardless of their status, can safely report concerns about other staff's behaviour.

Policies

While policies in and of themselves cannot protect against every eventuality, their development, monitoring and review at the very least promote awareness, identify risks and difficulties, and clarify priorities. Policies need to be clear in principle, widely agreed, possible to operationalise according to local need, and feasible in terms of resources. Managers and clinical governance representatives will need support in dissemination. Monitoring should be resourced centrally, for instance as trust-wide audit and quality projects, with sampling of certain areas and issues each year, supported by information technology and risk management systems.

Boundary transgressions can occur in many types of setting, both small and large. Because of the scandals of neglect and abuse in old institutions, especially of elderly and mentally handicapped persons, there was an assumption that 'community care' would provide greater safety. However, similar risks can arise with isolation, the lack of an 'open system', idiosyncratic practice, and power imbalances, which include lack of knowledge of how to react. A single central policy is unlikely to be sufficient, and will not command respect if it is obviously inapplicable – for instance general adult policies applied to children's wards or elderly day care. Local variations or elaborations need to be formulated and agreed in advance, rather than *ad hoc* non-standard 'exceptions' being accepted as necessary.

Patients and their carers should be actively involved in the setting up and review of policies and procedures. Regular opportunity for debate, involving patients and staff, may help raise consciousness and contribute to the development or modification of policies.

Staff disciplinary policies should cover not only expected standards of behaviour between staff and patients but also between staff and other staff or trainees. Characteristically, staff-to-staff behaviour policies have been developed in the business field and in universities, especially in the USA. The thinking behind them relates to the imbalance of power relationships and the potential for exploitation or unfairness. If expected behaviours are defined, then contraventions can be proceeded against using trust disciplinary policies, such as for 'harassment and bullying'.

Staff treating staff

This form of apparently harmless boundary breaking can in fact lead to harm and, occasionally, abuse. It is an example of the risk of 'dual relationship'. For instance, several of the Kerr/Haslam allegations (Department of Health, 2005*b*) related to nursing staff, even though they were formally registered as patients. A policy should be developed on this issue that bars examination or prescribing without formal referral and registration except in emergencies. All staff need to know this, so that they do not request help or respond to informal requests inappropriately.

Whistle-blowing

Inquiries have found that staff are often reluctant to express concern about colleagues because of embarrassment, fear of disbelief or retaliation, concerns about confidentiality, lack of clarity about whom to share the concern with, misplaced professional loyalty, and doubts about whether informing would make the matter better or worse. Health Service Circular 1999/198 (Department of Health, 1999) states that every NHS trust and health authority should have in place policies and procedures which comply with the Public Interest Disclosure Act 1998, and as a minimum include:

- guidance to help staff who have concerns about malpractice raise these reasonably and responsibly with the right parties
- the designation of a senior manager or non-executive director with specific responsibility for addressing concerns which need to be handled outside the usual management chain
- a clear commitment that staff concerns will be taken seriously and investigated
- an unequivocal guarantee that staff who raise concerns responsibly and reasonably will be protected against victimisation.

A 'whistle-blowing policy' should not primarily be intended to prevent staff going to the media with service concerns. Rather, it should facilitate the reporting of concerns about other staff. This could include the possibility of confidential discussion of concerns by staff, for instance by not giving the name at first, of either the complainant or of the person complained about. Someone outside the managerial line would need to be available for this, such as a non-executive director. There should also be provision for dealing with anonymous written complaints naming an individual, for instance that the appropriate manager should discuss the complaint with the individual named and maintain a note within the personnel record for a certain period, in case similar issues arise again. Of course, the possibility of false accusations, whether mistaken or malicious, must be kept in mind.

The organisation Public Concern at Work (PCaW; http://www.pcaw.co.uk) offers advice to individuals on how to raise concerns and to employers on good practice.

Sexual behaviour

A patient-centred policy is advisable, covering sexual behaviour between patients as well as between staff and patients, and could usefully also cover inappropriate behaviour towards staff by patients. This should refer to the 'vulnerable adults' policy and will need consultation with social services and the police.

Chaperones

A chaperone policy adaptable to all areas should be developed and resourced. If physical examination is intended, patients should be given information and offered a chaperone. The General Medical Council (2006) recommends that, wherever possible, the patient should be offered the security of having an impartial observer (a 'chaperone') present during an intimate examination. This would apply irrespective of the gender of doctor or patient. Clearly, a systematic approach to this would raise resource issues, but the safety of both patients and staff (who may be wrongly accused) would be promoted.

Response following an incident

Uncertainties about what to do following a reported sexual boundary transgression undoubtedly contributed to the extraordinary delays highlighted in the Kerr/Haslam Inquiry (Department of Health, 2005b). Trusts need to develop protocols in collaboration with local agencies, particularly social services and the police, and in consultation with their own legal service, following good practice guidance where possible. There will be many issues to consider, and it would be helpful to have thought about them in advance. Incidents should be regarded as likely to occur rather than unlikely. For instance, an 'untoward incident' policy may be relevant, as are the reporting requirements of the National Patient Safety Agency. Has the incident involved a minor? Has a crime possibly been committed under the Sexual Offences Act? If there is one known complainant, could other patients or staff also have been involved? If so, could and should they be alerted so that they would feel safe to come forward, and in a way that would not jeopardise any future legal action?

Policy non-compliance – investigations and disciplinary procedures

While there is no evidence that boundary transgressions are more prevalent among medical than other staff, it is clear from reported GMC cases that this is a significant issue. Taking action has been perceived to be difficult for a variety of reasons. Junior doctors may not themselves be clear about appropriate boundaries, and may not have been advised about the inherent vulnerabilities in the patient–doctor situation. They may not know whom to complain to or consult without fear of retaliation, such as bad references. There are uncertainties about what is or is not acceptable. Colleagues might be reluctant to believe accounts, or, worse, passively or actively collude. All of this also applies to other health professionals, who may wonder, suspect or know that improper conduct is taking place, but feel unable to challenge it. The GMC previously discouraged doctors from being negative about other doctors (see Chapter 4, p. 42); now this is phrased as 'you must not make malicious and unfounded criticisms of colleagues' and there is a duty to report concerns (General Medical Council, 2006).

Clinical governance is now clearly a trust responsibility. Guidance on medical disciplinary action is provided in *Maintaining High Professional Standards in the Modern NHS* (Department of Health, 2005a), while the National Clinical Assessment Service (NCAS) is available for consultation and assessment if necessary. Medical professional governance arrangements, such as appraisal and disciplinary mechanisms, are usually within the remit of the medical director, who has a management responsibility to the employing authority and also a professional duty in this respect to the GMC. The medical director's role is a key one, and will become more so especially in terms of liaison with the GMC as the role of 'responsible officer' in the revalidation process is clarified (General Medical Council, 2010).

Clinical practice

Assessment

Professional abuse inquiries have often found that risky situations arise when a physical examination is undertaken with unnecessary detail, such as demands for excessive undressing and inappropriate touching. This may be accompanied by inappropriately sexualised language and 'joking'. Services should have unambiguous protocols about what level of physical examination is required under different circumstances (e.g. admission, first out-patient attendance, emergency, home visits). In the development of such policies, consideration should be given to the possible interpretation of even a standard examination as intrusive, perhaps because of cultural beliefs and customs, or perhaps because of the patient's mental state.

Standard treatments

Clearly some treatments provide more opportunity for abuse than others. 'Medical' relaxation, produced for instance by benzodiazepines for an endoscopy or a one-to-one therapy session, can be risky both for opportunities for abuse and for confusion of the patient (which might lead to false accusations). Any 'touching' treatments may risk boundary confusion, as may even 'non-touch' one-to-one therapy especially if taking place in an isolated place or at an unusual time when few other staff are around.

Unorthodox treatments

Complementary therapies have been used by both medical and non-medical staff as if they are inherently safe and pleasant for the patient, because no medically prescribed medication is involved and irrespective of efficacy. However, 'novel and unusual treatments' were noted to be risk areas in the Kerr/Haslam report (Department of Health, 2005b), especially when they provided opportunities for unsupervised physical contact with vulnerable patients. Therapies such as massage, aromatherapy or acupuncture would fall into this group. In addition, 'non-touch' forms of therapy such as hypnosis or relaxation can also be risky for boundary transgression especially if done one-to-one.

Such therapies need tight clinical governance arrangements. Practitioners or their immediate supervisors should have special qualifications or training, belong to professional organisations, and be supervised externally or internally. Trusts should have evidence bases and protocols for the treatments they use and they should be aware of therapies being undertaken by all staff, through supervision, appraisals and job plans. A register of treatments is a useful mechanism for recording treatments and approved protocols; it could also include chaperone requirements, and specify levels of training and supervision requirements for each treatment.

A multidisciplinary protocol concerning the introduction or piloting of 'novel treatments' should be developed, which should include review of the evidence base. It is likely that some non-standard treatments will be used in research trials, and may be presented as being very special to the patient and not to be questioned by other staff, as reported by the Kerr/Haslam Inquiry.

Box 12.1 Unorthodox 'therapies'

Patients were made to feel special by being recruited for 'research' using a Kirlian camera to detect their 'hand auras'. Unorthodox 'therapies' were given, including 'Somlec' (weak electrical application to the temples, carbon dioxide inhalation for relaxation and unchaperoned whole-body massage). All these were for younger female patients only and often out of hours, in isolated hospital locations or private practice rooms.

Source: Kennedy (2006).

It is therefore essential that the local research ethics committee be aware of the risks and seek to reduce them. Trust and patient interests should be clearly represented on the committee.

Staff

The relevant points in relation to the management of staff issues to prevent boundary transgressions are summarised in Box 12.2.

Recruitment

Inquiries suggest that a number of sexual abuse incidents could be prevented if good recruitment practices were followed. There is a clear risk, evident from GMC cases, that doctors with a history of improper conduct may change employers without the new employers becoming aware of their history. While this has sometimes entailed moving from country to country, smaller moves have also succeeded. It would be implausible that candidates would reveal such problems at interview, so checking references fully is vital. A declaration on the application form about performance or disciplinary concerns would at least provide grounds for disciplinary action if the information turned out to be false. The Kerr/Haslam Inquiry recommended that one of the referees in any job application should be the consultant who conducts the applicant's appraisal, the clinical director or the medical director. References should be obtained from the three most recent employers and properly checked, for example by personally speaking to referees on a formal basis (not as an 'old friend').

Pre-employment police vetting should be undertaken to the highest possible level (such as via the Criminal Records Bureau disclosure system), as many if not most patients can be considered vulnerable. All staff, whether permanent, non-clinical, temporary or volunteer, should be checked if they have potential access to patients. When it is necessary to use agencies, only those that have police-checked their workers should be used.

Box 12.2 The management of medical staff and boundary transgression

- All medical staff should be alerted to boundary issues, with the different risks identified for each specialty area.
- All medical staff should be kept up to date on the latest recommendations of the GMC and the Royal Colleges on boundary issues.
- Consultant recruitment practice should be reviewed, especially verification of references, and a declaration required about previous disciplinary concerns.
- Job descriptions should be clear, and reviewed annually through the job planning mechanism.
- Professional membership should be a requirement.
- There should be an adviser from the relevant Royal College on the appointment panel.
- The above standards should also be met for honorary and locum consultant appointments.
- Annual appraisal needs to be comprehensively supported and include a 360-degree evaluation every 3 years.
- Clinical directors and other appraisers should be trained, especially in confronting performance or conduct issues.
- Consultant clinical practice needs to be open to audit and reflection by methods agreed with the appraiser as appropriate.
- University-linked post-holders should have an annual appraisal that includes a trust representative.

Job descriptions need to be full and clear on appointment so that it is easy to clarify later whether duties have been fulfilled.

Evidence of registration with the GMC is a condition of employment for medical staff. Professional membership is not legally compulsory but within the power of trusts to require and is recommended to help ensure standards. While foundation trusts have more flexibility in consultant appointments, there should be an advisor from the relevant Royal College to ensure a good quality of applicant. The trust should ensure its standards are also met for honorary consultant posts, and have appropriate representation on the academic consultant appointment committee if it is a university appointment. This should apply also to locum consultants appointed from outside the trust.

Performance

Supervision, appraisal and job planning systems must be systematically and effectively used for all clinical staff, irrespective of their status. Consultants should undergo formal annual appraisal, often by their clinical director. To ensure standards, appraisers should be trained, samples of documentation audited, and a robust 360-degree process included which requires comments from a sample of colleagues and patients. The last should help to clarify issues of probity and health, which otherwise are covered essentially by self-declaration or what is known personally by the appraiser.

The trust needs to support appraisal by ensuring time, appraiser training, and relevant activity, incident and complaints data. The training of appraisers should cover how to approach difficult issues, including boundary violation, and all types of therapy undertaken should be agreed and noted within the appraisal documentation. Evidence of continued professional development (CPD) is required for appraisal and is most easily obtained by psychiatrists by registering with the Royal College of Psychiatrists, meeting with a peer group to discuss the goals, and annually sending in evidence for certification. The appraiser also discusses with the appraisee work goals and any remediation or learning necessary and should review these annually.

If the appraisal raises concerns about practice, the medical director should be informed, in order to take any necessary action, which could be internal, or could take the form of referral to the NCAS or the GMC. If a consultant's practice is impaired, this is often due to poor health and/or long-standing personality characteristics affecting judgement. The usual first-line corrective actions, such as talking the issue over, may not succeed. Nonetheless, in the past, poor practice could go entirely unchallenged. If the doctor is willing to discuss the issues, then various actions are possible. The NCAS can advise, mediate and if necessary formally assess the doctor. Serious performance problems, including those due to poor health, especially when not accepted by the doctor, can be referred to the GMC, which will be happy to discuss any issue informally first.

'Clinical supervision' is an ambiguous term but supervision systems for senior clinicians should be considered. Some trusts do this through CPD peer groups, but other models are possible. 'Clinical supervision' has a number of different meanings to health professionals and *Safeguarding Patients* (Department of Health, 2007) does not require this of consultant psychiatrists in terms of making their practice less autonomous than consultants of other specialties. Nevertheless, open and reflective practice is both safer and desirable, is quite usual clinically, and can be achieved by a number of methods.

The management process for staff who are employed by a university but who also engage in direct work with trust patients can be ambiguous. The Follett report (Follett & Paulson-Ellis, 2001) recommended that honorary consultant staff with university appointments should undergo appraisal for their clinical commitments in a similar way to those employed by the NHS, probably with two appraisers, one each from the trust and university. There should be clear documentation of this process, and agreement as to which party should hold the personnel records, receive and investigate complaints, be responsible for disciplinary action and so on. There also need to be agreements about the job plan and service or research expectations. While these need to be detailed on appointment, changes are likely to be necessary and would need negotiation, for which clear mechanisms are important.

There may be similar difficulties with doctors working part time for different employers, partly in private practice, or even across several sites, with ambiguity about who is primarily responsible. Locum doctors may also fall 'under the radar' unless arrangements are clear.

Staff training

Training is an essential part of any policy for dealing with abuse. This should not be a one-off event, as different types of presentation will be appropriate for different groups at different times. However, opportunities arise in induction and risk management as well as in the usual educational and training programmes, multidiscipline as well as single discipline. As relevant policies are introduced or amended, training opportunities will naturally arise with their dissemination.

All medical staff should be updated on the latest recommendations of the GMC, the Committee for Healthcare Regulatory Excellence and relevant Royal Colleges.

In addition, managers and clinical directors responsible for investigations and inquiries should have training in disciplinary procedures and investigation methods.

Patient/service user issues

A repeated refrain within inquiries is that patients/service users who have been abused are often unclear about who they should complain to, uncertain of their grounds and vulnerable to threats such as withdrawal of service. As with any form of sexual harassment or abuse, there is likely to be shame and embarrassment, a fear of disbelief and a reluctance to make formal complaints and allegations in writing, in public and repeatedly – conditions which have often been demanded before investigations are pursued. Mental health service users may be particularly vulnerable because of a history of previous abuse, reluctance to be known to be using mental health services, and fear of their story being discounted as a consequence. Although some allegations of boundary transgression may be inaccurate misperceptions or even malicious on the part of the patient, such possibilities should not preclude the offer of serious and respectful attention.

Information

Letters, explanations, leaflets and notices should all be used to clarify what patients should expect in terms of examination, questions, investigations or treatment. Ideally, these will be produced or modified in consultation

147

with patient and voluntary groups to ensure their comprehensibility and acceptability for the various settings.

If physical examination is intended, patients should be given information and offered a chaperone. Patients need to have a clear understanding of the nature of the examination being undertaken, the implications and their rights to a chaperone in all circumstances, not just where an intimate examination is being undertaken.

Patients and carers should be told about how to:

- comment on the service
- raise a concern
- make a formal complaint
- access advocacy services and other agencies offering assistance.

New patients especially need to know what to expect in terms of questions likely to be asked, examinations and investigations made, and entitlement to chaperones. The same applies to new forms of assessment or treatment being offered. Guidance documents have been developed by the Council for Healthcare Regulatory Excellence (see http://www.chre.org.uk).

Patient complaints

From the Kerr/Haslam Inquiry it is evident that patients need to be able to approach someone informally to discuss concerns before committing themselves to a formal complaint. While patient advice and liaison services (PALS) and complaints department staff certainly should be trained to help, any staff may be the recipients of such information and need to know how to act (Box 12.3). Often reasons given for the receiving member of staff not taking things further are that the patient did not wish to make a written or public statement, or be involved in an investigation, whether from the trust, the GMC, social services or the police, and did not consent to the breaking of confidentiality. However, there are limits to confidentiality requirements where safety is involved. Equally, patients should not have to undergo repeated questioning. This is the sort of issue which staff should be able to discuss with a designated person outside their own management line if necessary.

Support and counselling

Once a formal complaint has been made, the complainant may need further support, both for his or her own well-being and to facilitate the effectiveness of any inquiry. While practical and immediate steps may be the priority, subsequently patients who have been subject to sexual abuse by staff may wish for access to independent psychotherapeutic treatment. The voluntary agency Witness (previously POPAN; Prevention of Professional Abuse Network) has been a useful source of advice on this (now superseded by the Clinic for Boundary Studies, http://www.professionalboundaries.org.uk).

> **Box 12.3** The difficulties of complaining
>
> 'A minority of patients divulged the abuse at the time to a general practitioner, a psychiatric nurse, or another psychiatrist. Most professionals did no more than pass on gossip to colleagues and alter referral habits. Patients said they had expected much more decisive action. Ironically, concern was expressed about Kerr on one occasion to his wife, also a consultant psychiatrist, and on another occasion to Haslam. The very few patients who submitted formal written complaints all declined to take part in any formal disciplinary proceedings – sometimes after intimidation by the psychiatrist concerned ("No one will believe you against the word of a consultant").'
>
> Source: Kennedy (2006).

Other clinical governance methods

Monitoring, risk and quality

Sexual boundary transgressions between staff and patients are probably not infrequent, although in the past they may often have been overlooked. From the risk management point of view, they should be looked upon as high risk, with major impact in terms of cost, which could include court cases, inquiry costs and damage to a trust's reputation. The advantage of formalising consideration of this possibility is that it involves regular thinking about prevention and methods of monitoring. Patient complaints are usually monitored but may not be the best indicator of what is happening. In addition, staff may report other staff, but this too has limitations as an indicator as, for instance, agency and locum staff may be reported to their direct employer or just not be used again.

Consideration could be given to making reports of 'untoward incidents' contain a relevant data category. As incidents are reported, internal inquiries should identify and address outstanding policy and training needs in the area of sexual abuse. Audit and quality systems could also be used to improve clinical practice. For example, an audit to establish the extent of use of 'unorthodox' treatments might be revealing, and lead to ideas on how to establish related quality standards.

Occupational health and staff support

The occupational health and staff support services have dual roles in providing a service to the trust and to those who consult them. They are likely to hear about employment-related causes of stress, including incidents of bullying and harassment, and also occasionally of suspected patient abuse. Their staff should therefore be knowledgeable about boundary transgression, and explain the limits of confidentiality to their clients. Regular (at least annual) reporting of types of issues raised, with a systematic format, would help to keep the trust informed.

The medical manager's role

The medical director can have a key role in improving standards across an organisation by accepting that boundary violations are a serious issue for doctors, and hence for all staff. Monitoring methods are frequently present but not well used. 'Quality' and 'complaints' may be seen as issues for the lead nurse, 'research ethics' for the academics, 'risk' for the finance department and 'whistle-blowing' for the unions and the human resources department. The medical director's skills are likely to be challenged in this area, as he or she may well face reluctance, suspicion and opposition. It is not surprising that 'dealing with difficult colleagues' is a popular training course, and it is wise to look for allies within the organisation as well as support and training outside.

References

Council for Healthcare Regulatory Excellence (2008) *Clear Sexual Boundaries between Healthcare Professionals and Patients: Responsibilities of Healthcare Professionals.* CHRE.

Department of Health (1999) *The Public Interest Disclosure Act 1998* (HSC 1999/198). Department of Health.

Department of Health (2005a) *Maintaining High Professional Standards in the Modern NHS.* Department of Health.

Department of Health (2005b) *The Kerr/Haslam Inquiry.* TSO (The Stationery Office).

Department of Health (2007) *Safeguarding Patients: The Government's Response to the Recommendations of the Shipman Inquiry's Fifth Report and to the Recommendations of the Ayling, Neale and Kerr/Haslam Inquiries*, pp. 54–61. TSO (The Stationery Office).

Follett, B. & Paulson-Ellis, M. (2001) *A Review of Appraisal, Disciplinary and Reporting Arrangements of Senior NHS and University Staff with Academic and Clinical Duties* (Follett report). Department of Education and Skills

General Medical Council (2006) *Maintaining Boundaries.* GMC. Available online at http://www.gmc-uk.org/guidance/ethical_guidance/maintaining_boundaries.asp (accessed 18 July 2010).

General Medical Council (2010) Revalidation – responsible officer. http://www.gmc-uk.org/doctors/revalidation/responsible_officer.asp (accessed 25 July 2010).

Home Office (2004) *Working with the Sexual Offences Act 2003.* Home Office.

Kennedy, P. (2006) The Kerr/Haslam Inquiry into sexual abuse of patients by psychiatrists. *Psychiatric Bulletin*, **30**, 204–206.

CHAPTER 13

Dealing with offending doctors: sanctions and remediation

Pete Snowden

Overview

This chapter is primarily concerned with the range of sanctions – criminal, employment and regulatory – that can be used to deal with doctors who transgress professional boundaries. It also looks at prevention, as well as the remediation (where this is thought to be possible) and possible return to work of doctors who offend. Two case vignettes are used to illustrate the issues. As with much of the rest of this book, the focus is on sexual misconduct and offending.

Introduction

Being a doctor does not make a person a law-abiding model citizen. Doctors commit offences outside of professional practice, including sexual offences. Male (and, less frequently, female) doctors do so for similar reasons to others in society, and this should not be surprising.

A second group of doctors behaves in a sexually inappropriate manner with patients. The data from North America (Gartrell *et al*, 1986; Morrison & Wickersham, 1998; Bloom *et al*, 1999) and Australia (Quadrio, 1996) suggest that 3–10% of doctors admit to some form of sexual involvement with a patient. For each doctor there may be a number of patient victims. For example, it was estimated that around 70 women claimed to have been sexually assaulted by the consultant psychiatrist William Kerr (see Box 6.2, p. 66).

Gabbard (1999) has proposed a psychodynamic categorisation for doctors who behave inappropriately in a sexual manner and/or who offend. Evidence received by the Kerr/Haslam Inquiry (Department of Health, 2005) suggested that for doctors or therapists who sexually abuse patients, the most common type is the 'predatory psychopath' (see also Box 8.4, p. 99). Abel & Osborn (1999), in a North American study of cases of professional misconduct, found that 20% of the sample had a paraphilia (sexual deviation) which extended into their professional practice. A simpler method of categorisation (see Box 13.1) is to consider where the sexual misconduct/offending takes place, and with whom, as this helps in decisions on sanctions and the feasibility of remediation (Box 13.2).

Whatever the subtype, and however the misconduct itself is dealt with, the nature of these worrying misbehaviours means that there will be always be concern about future risks to patients. The guiding principle in the handling of sexual misconduct and offending is that patient safety must be paramount, not the professional career of the practitioner.

For each doctor, sexual misconduct and offending may result in one or all of the following:

- criminal sanctions
- employment sanctions
- regulatory sanctions.

Box 13.1 Categorisation by location of the offence

- *Outside professional practice.* A doctor under the influence of alcohol sexually assaults a woman outside a nightclub.
- *At the workplace but not against patients.* A doctor accesses illegal pornography on the internet from an office using a workplace computer.
- *Against patients.* A psychiatrist commits a sexual assault or indecent act in the setting of individual psychotherapy.
- *A mixed presentation.* More than one of the above.

Box 13.2 Case vignette 1: categorisation of offences by place and those involved

When Dr X was a young adolescent he experienced a failed attempt at intercourse, which he found embarrassing and humiliating. At around the same time he was seen by a group of girls urinating behind a tree in a local park. He remembers them laughing at him as they ran off. He described these two events as upsetting formative experiences which he recognised were linked to what became regular episodes of indecent (masturbatory) exposure. He estimated that there were hundreds of similar episodes during his student years.

As a junior on-call doctor he would 'set up' situations where he would expose himself to nurses in hospital residential accommodation. He was spoken to about his behaviour but escaped serious censure.

He was arrested and convicted of indecent exposure for a series of episodes that occurred outside the hospital where he worked. There was never any evidence of misconduct with patients.

Criminal sanctions

In June 2006 the Home Office updated the 1986 guidance (Home Office, 2006) for police forces for what is termed the Notifiable Occupations Scheme. Doctors are one of the professional groups covered by this scheme, which deals with those occupations that 'carry special trust or responsibility, in which the public interest in the disclosure of conviction and other information by the police generally outweighs the normal duty of confidentiality owed to the individual'. In the UK the General Medical Council (GMC) will be informed of any police investigation, arrest, caution, reprimand or warning, and any conviction for recordable offences (any offence under UK law where the police are allowed to keep records on the Police National Database). The GMC will ask the doctor who his or her employer is and will then inform the employer directly by letter of the situation. If the matter is still sub judice (arrested but not charged) the employer is told of the fact of the arrest, and no further information is supplied until conviction or acquittal. In urgent cases or risky situations (for example where there is concern about possible harm to children or vulnerable adults) the police can directly inform the employer as well as the regulatory body.

For independent practitioners, where the risks cannot be managed locally the case can be dealt with quickly by an interim orders panel of the GMC.

Employment sanctions

In 2003 the Department of Health issued the document *Maintaining High Professional Standards in the NHS: A Framework for the Initial Handling of Concerns About Doctors and Dentists in the NHS*. One of the key changes was the abolition of the distinction between personal and professional misconduct; both are viewed as disciplinary matters for the National Health Service (NHS) employer, rather than an external body.

When an employer has information that raises serious concerns about a practitioner (for example from the GMC after a doctor has been arrested) there is a responsibility to consider restrictions on practice to protect patients, or in the public interest.

The sexual misconduct of a doctor may well be first recognised by hospital staff, and be responded to by management for those doctors who offend in the workplace, and who are employed in a managed environment in the NHS or an independent hospital. Internet surveillance systems supported by the majority of these organisations will trigger an adverse report to management when banned or illegal websites are accessed (Box 13.3).

The employer response can be immediate exclusion from work while disciplinary actions are triggered. The employer will in these cases also inform the GMC.

Box 13.3 Case vignette 2, part I: inappropriate websites

A consultant began to access sexually inappropriate websites depicting pornography and violence. For many years he had spent varying amounts of time on similar websites using his home computer. He began to use his hospital office computer during a stressful period in his professional and domestic life. Within a week he was called to meet his medical director and was informed that he would be immediately excluded from work.

An immediate exclusion from work is time limited, usually for up to a maximum of 2 weeks. The manager making the decision will set up an investigation and decide whether it is necessary to consider formal exclusion to protect patients, or in the public interest. If immediate exclusion needs to be extended beyond 2 weeks, it must be reviewed before the end of every 4-week period. The total length of time of this process, and the work of any investigation panel, will be governed by the nature of the misconduct and the criminal justice process for those doctors who have been charged with an offence (Box 13.4).

The role of the National Clinical Assessment Service

The National Clinical Assessment Service (NCAS) was set up in 2001 to help the NHS deal better with the performance of doctors, mainly because of the frequent use of prolonged suspension from work. It receives 'referrals' (requests for help) from a variety of sources, but the great majority are from employers – hospital and community trusts and primary care trusts and their equivalents across the UK. The aim is to advise on management of the situation, proceeding to full formal assessment of the practitioner if necessary. Telephone advice is sufficient in about 60% of cases.

The NCAS has recently reported on its first 8 years of cases (National Clinical Assessment Service, 2009). There were 4692 referrals of individual practitioners, 269 assessments begun and 236 assessments completed.

Box 13.4 Case vignette 2, part II: exclusion and investigation

The police investigation found no evidence of material which would warrant anything more than a police caution, and the GMC was informed. The employing NHS trust at this point was able to complete its own investigation. During the whole process, which lasted a number of months, the consultant was excluded from work, but had been referred by his general practitioner to a psychotherapist.

It notes that: 'Psychiatry, obstetrics and gynaecology (O&G) and general medical practice have noticeably more referrals than might be expected from their workforce size'. However, for psychiatry there were relatively fewer cases that proceeded to assessment, although this finding may be affected by more referrals being made of non-UK-qualified, non-white doctors, of whom psychiatry has a larger proportion. There were fewer referrals of women than the workforce size would predict.

Since 2007, case concerns have been logged by category. Analysis of 1472 cases shows that 33% were categorised as misconduct. The other categories were clinical difficulties (54%), governance/safety issues (36%), other behavioural difficulties (29%), health problems (24%) and work environment influences (11%). More than one concern could be identified, with about 16% of cases involving misconduct alone, the largest distinct concern category.

It can be seen from Table 13.1 that sexual issues are of frequent concern, but other disturbances of the relationship between the doctor, other staff and patients are common.

An NCAS performance assessment results in recommendations for the practitioner and the referring organisation. In the majority of cases a remediation programme is proposed, following the principles of the *Back on Track* document (National Clinical Assessment Service, 2006; see also below).

Regulatory sanctions

Regulatory sanctions are the province of the General Medical Council (GMC). These processes are separate from disciplinary procedures undertaken by a doctor's employer and from criminal proceedings. The role of the GMC is discussed fully in Chapter 16. Here, it is sufficient to note that there is a

Table 13.1 Misconduct concerns dealt with by the National Clinical Assessment Service (NCAS) (source: NCAS, 2009).

Misconduct sub-concern (sexual categories in italic)	Percentage*
Theft, fraud, financial	20
Driving under the influence of drugs or alcohol	1
Other misuse of drugs or alcohol	5
Breach of confidentiality	4
Inappropriate sexual relationship with patient	3
Other sexual misconduct	10
Assault/threatening behaviour	7
Bullying/harassment/discrimination	12
Other personal misconduct towards patient or staff	16
Use of illegal pornography	2
Use of legal pornography at work	2
Other misuse of resources/equipment	9

*9% not classified in source

considerable range of outcomes that may follow a process of investigation by the GMC, which include:

- not proceeding with a complaint
- referral back to local procedures
- voluntary undertakings
- interim action to protect patients, such as conditions on or suspension of registration
- a decision that fitness-to-practise is impaired.

In the last instance, the GMC's sanctions include warning, conditions on or suspension of registration, and erasure.

Erasure

The most serious sanction is to erase a doctor from the Register. Sexual misconduct is one of the three areas of serious concern (the others being dishonesty and failures in treatment/care) which can lead to this sanction. A doctor erased from the Register must wait 5 years before applying to be restored. The Privy Council has upheld erasure decisions in cases of serious misconduct despite strong mitigation such as ill-health and has stated:

The public, and in particular female patients, must have confidence in the medical profession whatever their state of health might be. The conduct as found proved … undoubtedly undermines such confidence and a severe sanction was inevitable. Their Lordships are satisfied that erasure was neither unreasonable, excessive nor disproportionate but necessary in the public interest. (Privy Council, 2002)

Where a doctor is convicted of a sexual offence, where there is an abuse of trust, or where the doctor has to register as a sex offender, erasure has been judged to be an appropriate sanction. A conviction for child pornography is viewed by the GMC as a matter of grave concern because it involves a fundamental breach of patients' trust in doctors. A conviction of this nature in UK law will lead to sex offender registration. In these cases no doctor can have unrestricted GMC registration, and contact with any patient group is questionable (General Medical Council, 2009). The likelihood is that the most appropriate sanction is erasure in such cases.

Referral to medical and lay case examiners

Where the conviction does not fall within the list of convictions for serious offences which would trigger an automatic referral to a Fitness to Practise (FTP) panel, the case is referred to case examiners, who have available the following decisions:

- conclude the case with no further action
- issue a warning on future conduct

- refer the case to a FTP panel
- ask the doctor to agree to undertakings.

Undertakings

When an investigation committee or the case examiners are satisfied that there is no prospect of determining that a doctor's fitness to practise is impaired, yet further action is necessary, but a warning is thought not to be enough, then 'voluntary undertakings' may be deemed a proportionate and appropriate response to protect patients and the public and to address the concerns about the practitioner (Box 13.5). The doctor must accept the undertakings and disclose them to his or her employer, must show insight into the problems and be willing to accept remediation.

Undertakings may include restrictions on a doctor's practice or behaviour, or a commitment to undergo medical supervision or retraining. Undertakings will usually be disclosed to the doctor's employer and to any other enquirer, and are published on the GMC website list of Registered Medical Practitioners.

There are three types of undertaking:

- those relating to the treatment of a doctor's underlying health condition
- those relating to the need to remedy deficiencies in clinical performance
- those relating to day-to-day practice.

Council for Healthcare Regulatory Excellence

The Council for Healthcare Regulatory Excellence (CHRE) is now the overarching regulator in the United Kingdom and may refer decisions to the High Court if they are 'unduly lenient and do not protect the public' (see Council for Healthcare Regulatory Excellence, 2010, section 3.1).

Box 13.5 Case vignette 2, part III: undertakings

The GMC took the view that limitations on registration were unnecessary but the consultant agreed to a number of undertakings in order to maintain registration. These included seeing a GMC supervisor on a regular basis, continuing with the psychotherapy and any other treatment to meet his risk needs, and informing any future employer about the nature of his computer misuse so that robust monitoring systems could be put in place. However, his employer found on investigation that there had been a serious breach of hospital policy and he was dismissed from his post.

Prevention

In the USA, the Federation of State Medical Boards has recommended that the state medical boards (which license medical practitioners) should have in place:

- proactive strategies to improve medical education about professional boundaries
- early intervention at medical school and residency programmes when sexual misconduct is reported
- educational courses for licensed doctors.

Educational courses on this subject attract continuing medical education (CME) points. Spickard *et al* (2002, 2008), from Vanderbilt University, Nashville, describe a 3-day 'maintaining proper boundaries' course with a combined didactic approach and guided introspection. The course leaders are all addiction trained and experienced in working with clients who present with minimisation, rationalisation and denial. The Physician Assessment and Clinical Education (PACE) Program (http://www.paceprogram.ucsd.edu/cpd.aspx) at the University of California, San Diego, offers a professional boundaries programme to assist doctors to:

- develop a greater understanding of the multiple issues and factors that lead to sexual harassment and sexual misconduct in the workplace
- increase knowledge and understanding of the impact of sexual harassment and sexual misconduct on victims and work
- increase insight into personal attitudes and paradigms about work, power, self-esteem, gender and cultural factors, and issues of sexuality
- clarify values and boundaries
- improve coping skills
- develop appropriate work-based behaviours.

There are other examples of boundary education programmes in the USA (see for example http://www.professionalboundaries.com/index.php). However, there has been no evaluation of the efficacy of an educational approach in preventing boundary violations.

In the UK, education of medical students and physicians on professional boundaries, boundary crossing, boundary violations and the risks of sexual misconduct has been generally poor (see Chapter 3). The Council for Healthcare Regulatory Excellence has published three guidance documents on sexual boundaries (see http://www.chre.org.uk/satellite/133, and Chapter 15). This comprised guidance for FTP panels, general advice for regulators, and a report on education and training (Council for Healthcare Regulatory Excellence, 2008*a–c*). It is argued in the last that good education and training are important parts of a strategy to prevent health professionals from breaching sexual boundaries with patients or their carers, and that this should begin in student training. There are currently no educational providers of this type of training in the UK.

Remediation

Although in the USA (as in the UK) there have been concerns about the return to work of *any* doctor who offends sexually, some physicians have been allowed to return to a modified form of practice (often not in their previous role), with appropriate supervision, monitoring and safety measures in place, *after* the doctor has undertaken a course of treatment or education. This process is often described as remediation. Whether remediation is a realistic option is dependent on the type of sexual misconduct, the criminal and regulatory sanctions, the employer response, and the attitude of the professional concerned.

In some cases, despite protestations from the offending doctor who wishes to be retrained or treated, this may not be supported by the GMC because of the seriousness of the case and the importance of maintaining public safety and confidence in the profession.

In other cases, where the doctor has limitations on practice through GMC sanctions or has had sanctions removed to allow a reintegration into work, the employer may still decide no longer to employ the practitioner. A remediation process is a much more difficult enterprise if the doctor is not working in a managed environment.

Where it is believed to be potentially realistic for a particular clinician to be helped by a remedial programme (and where there is employer support) there will first have to be a comprehensive assessment of the sexual misconduct. This will need to be undertaken by a psychiatrist or psychologist experienced in the field.

The next step, before any remediation process is embarked upon, is to consider whether there is evidence of:

- insight into the nature of the sexual offending/misconduct on a personal and professional level
- acceptance that a serious problem exists
- empathy, or a capacity for empathy, with the victim
- commitment and genuine willingness to change.

Embarking on remediation is not realistic without insight, a capacity for empathy and commitment to change (Box 13.6).

Much of the experience in this field comes from North America and Australia. The approach in the USA (Swiggart *et al*, 2002) is for psychological treatment to take place if the licence to practise is not removed, and where there is evidence of a sexual disorder. Abel & Osborn (1999) and others (Irons & Schneider, 1999) have used a cognitive–behavioural treatment programme for professionals. The approach is similar to the treatment

> **Box 13.6** Case vignette 2, part IV: remediation
>
> The consultant continued to see his psychotherapist, and recognised that therapy would be a long-term process. However, he wanted to get back into work. He had enough insight to realise that he would not be able to work again in a consultant role, so he applied for supervised positions. He was honest about the recent difficulties and the reason for parting company with his previous NHS employer at interview and found appropriate employment. He does not have his own office or a work computer for his sole use.

of other offenders. Psychodynamic approaches also have been described (Gabbard, 1999). However, there are no follow-up data on whether treatment is effective in preventing further episodes of sexual misconduct.

When there is no evidence of an underlying sexual disorder, an educational programme is recommended. An example is the CME course described by Spickard *et al* (2002, 2008) in Nashville, which does accept physicians with sexual boundary violations referred by the state licensing board. The California PACE programme also accepts on its professional boundaries course doctors who:

- have had a complaint or grievance against them for sexual harassment in the workplace
- are at risk of losing their job, practice, privileges, or licence owing to allegations of sexual misconduct
- are on probation or suspension while under investigation
- need to meet court, state board or employer recommendations for sexual harassment/misconduct prevention training.

Although these are all educational programmes in design, the descriptions in published material suggest that there is a therapeutic component.

The Vanderbilt University, Nashville, research group (Swiggart *et al*, 2008) has also developed a screening tool which is said to show some early and encouraging results in identifying physicians at risk of boundary violations. This might also have utility for monitoring purposes.

A group in Zurich (Tschan, 2007; Tschan & Schoener, 2008) has described a remedial boundary programme ('modular offence focused intervention') for doctors who have presented with professional sexual misconduct. The goals of this programme are to re-establish professional competence, to solve the underlying problems in order to prevent relapse, and to follow up with monitoring. After a detailed assessment, including whether the doctor is suitable for the programme, a rehabilitation plan and treatment contract are developed. The next stage is boundary training, followed by job re-entry and monitoring.

In the UK there are no similar educational remedial training opportunities. The general opinion has been that in considering remediation of offending doctors, educational remedial training is not suitable unless there are other areas of clinical or behavioural deficiencies that require attention. This may not be correct and experience outside the UK suggests that an educational approach may be worthwhile.

Returning to work

There are no published studies on returning to work following remedial treatment or an educational approach. Even if the doctor has undergone successful treatment and/or education and is thought to be safe to recommence supervised practice, there may be many other hurdles to overcome. There will need to be detailed consideration of the work environment, the work expected of the doctor, and a gradual reintroduction plan in place. Colleagues may also need help and support in accepting the doctor back into the workplace. The elements of restoring doctors back into safe professional practice are described in the National Clinical Assessment Service's (2006) document *Back on Track* on restoring doctors and dentists to safe professional practice. This deals with doctors returning to work following local or national performance procedures because of health concerns, clinical practice concerns or behaviour, after these have been successfully dealt with. While not aimed at doctors who sexually offend or who have presented with boundary violations, the guiding principles remain relevant in these situations also:

- Clinical governance and patient safety are paramount.
- A comprehensive and realistic approach to address the needs of the individual and employing organisation is essential.
- The process should be fair and transparent, and as far as possible the confidentiality of the doctor should be respected, but patient consent to receiving care from a practitioner undertaking a return-to-work programme is required.
- Ongoing and consistent support is required.
- The framework developed for the doctor should address the possibility of failure and not just success.

In Canada there is some guidance available on return to work following sexual misconduct or sexual offending. The College of Physicians and Surgeons of Alberta (1992) has developed a common-sense position set out in *Guidelines for Considering Reinstatement of a Medical Licence or the Lifting of Suspension of a Licence to Practise following Sexual Exploitation of a Patient*. In consideration of an application for reinstatement of a licence to practise, where a doctor has been found to have sexually exploited a patient, then this will be considered only where there is evidence that:

- There is a clear diagnosis of the physician's condition.
- There is no evidence of psychopathy in the physician.

- The physician has admitted guilt without external pressure.
- The physician has shown a capacity for guilt and remorse.
- The physician has demonstrated the ability to self-report feelings honestly.
- All clinical work will be under supervision.
- The physician will not be able to perform psychotherapy.
- Reinstatement will be in the public interest.
- The probability of a repeat occurrence of patient abuse is virtually nil.
- The physician is prepared to enter into a contract for supervision.

The importance of close monitoring and supervision as part of a return-to-work programme cannot be overemphasised.

Conclusion

Much of the research on offending doctors and remediation comes from outside the UK. It is clear from these publications that there is some optimism that remediation can be a realistic option. Perhaps in the UK there is a less-forgiving culture; high-profile cases where doctors have sexually abused patients have reinforced the message that patient safety is paramount and not the doctor's career. The way that such cases are dealt with through criminal, regulatory and employment processes probably explains why little effort has gone into remediation approaches. However, there is arguably a need to better educate doctors on professional boundaries, boundary crossing and boundary transgression as a preventive measure. For the less-serious cases a structured remediation approach would be worth exploring.

References

Abel, G. & Osborn, C. A. (1999) Cognitive–behavioural treatment of sexual misconduct. In *Physician Sexual Misconduct* (eds J. D. Bloom, C. C. Nadelson & M. T. Notman), pp. 225–246. American University Press.

Bloom, J. D., Nadelson, C. C. & Notman, M. T. (1999) *Physician Sexual Misconduct*. American University Press.

College of Physicians and Surgeons of Alberta (1992) *Guidelines for Considering Reinstatement of a Medical Licence or the Lifting of Suspension of a Licence to Practise following Sexual Exploitation of a Patient*. CPSA.

Council for Healthcare Regulatory Excellence (2008a) *Clear Sexual Boundaries Between Healthcare Professionals and Patients: Guidance for Fitness to Practise Panels*. CHRE. Available online at http://www.chre.org.uk/_img/pics/library/0809_harmonising_sanctions_chre_view_FINAL_3.pdf (accessed June 2010).

Council for Healthcare Regulatory Excellence (2008b) *Clear Sexual Boundaries Between Healthcare Professionals and Patients: Responsibilities of Healthcare Professionals*. CHRE. Available online at http://www.chre.org.uk/satellite/133 (accessed June 2010).

Council for Healthcare Regulatory Excellence (2008c) *Learning About Sexual Boundaries Between Healthcare Professionals and Patients: A Report on Education and Training*. CHRE. Available online at http://www.chre.org.uk/satellite/133 (accessed June 2010).

Council for Healthcare Regulatory Excellence (2010) *Performance Review Report 2009/10: Enhancing Public Protection Through Improved Regulation*. TSO (The Stationery Office). Available online at http://www.chre.org.uk/_img/pics/library/100701_Performance_review_report_2009-10.pdf (accessed June 2010).

Department of Health (2003) *Maintaining High Professional Standards in the NHS: A Framework for the Initial Handling of Concerns About Doctors and Dentists in the NHS*. Department of Health.

Department of Health (2005) *The Kerr/Haslam Inquiry*. TSO (The Stationery Office).

Gabbard, G. O. (1999) Psychodynamic approaches to physician sexual misconduct. In *Physician Sexual Misconduct* (eds J. D. Bloom, C. C. Nadelson & M. T. Notman), pp. 205–223. American University Press.

Gartrell, N., Herman, J., Olarte, S., *et al* (1986) Psychiatrist–patient sexual contact: results of a national survey. I: Prevalence. *American Journal of Psychiatry*, **143**, 1126–1131.

General Medical Council (2009) *Indicative Sanctions Guidance*. GMC.

Home Office (2006) Notifiable occupations scheme: revised guidance for police. 1 April; Circular 6/2006. Home Office.

Irons, R. & Schneider, J. P. (1999) *The Wounded Healer: Addiction Sensitive Approach*. Jason Aronson.

Morrison J. & Wickersham, P. (1998) Physicians disciplined by a state medical board. *JAMA*, **279**, 1889–1893.

National Clinical Assessment Service (2006) *Back on Track. Restoring Doctors and Dentists to Safe Professional Practice*. Framework Document. NCAS. Available online at http://www.ncas.npsa.nhs.uk/EasySiteWeb/GatewayLink.aspx?alId=7966 (accessed June 2010).

National Clinical Assessment Service (2009) *NCAS Casework: The First Eight Years*. Available online at http://www.ncas.npsa.nhs.uk/news/first-eight-years (accessed June 2010).

Privy Council (2002) Appeal No. 69 of 2001, Dr Mohamed Shaker Haikel v. the General Medical Council. Available online at http://www.privy-council.org.uk/output/Page51.asp (accessed June 2010).

Quadrio, C. (1996) Sexual abuse in therapy: gender issues. *Australian and New Zealand Journal of Psychiatry*, **30**, 124–133.

Spickard, W. A., Swiggart, W., Manley, G., *et al* (2002) A continuing education course for physicians who cross boundaries. *Sexual Addiction and Compulsivity*, **9**, 33–42.

Spickard, W. A., Swiggart, W., Manley, G., *et al* (2008) A CME course to improve sexual boundaries. *Bulletin of the Menninger Clinic*, **72**, 38–53.

Swiggart, W., Starr, K., Finlayson, R., *et al* (2002) Sexual boundaries and physicians: overview and educational approach to the problem. *Sexual Addiction and Compulsivity*, **9**, 139–148.

Swiggart, W., Feurer, I. D., Samenow, C., *et al* (2008) Sexual Boundary Violation Index: a validation study. *Sexual Addiction and Compulsivity*, **15**, 176–190.

Tschan, W. (2007) Rehabilitation of offenders after PSM (professional sexual misconduct). *Proceedings of Postgraduate Training Meeting*. NSW Branch of RANZCP, Sydney. 7 March. Available online at http://www.bsgp.ch/userdocs/Sydney%202007%20pdf.pdf (accessed June 2010).

Tschan, W. & Schoener, G. (2008) Innovations in the evaluation of professionals who engage in boundary violations. Issue Workshop: 161st American Psychiatric Association Meeting, 3–8 May. Available online at http://www.bsgp.ch/pages/english.php (accessed June 2010).

CHAPTER 14

Defending doctors: the protection society's experience

Andrew Pickering

Overview

This chapter looks at the experience of a medico-legal adviser at the Medical Protection Society (MPS) in dealing with doctors who find themselves accused of boundary violations. It reviews the types of behaviour that lead to accusations of boundary violations and the various forums in which they may be raised (the situation known as multiple jeopardy). The chapter looks at some data available from cases with which the MPS has assisted and attempts to identify gross patterns. Then advice from regulatory bodies and the MPS's experience are summarised in order to help doctors avoid such allegations. A fictionalised case example has been included to illustrate the wide-reaching effects of an allegation on a doctor's professional and personal life.

Introduction

The Medical Protection Society (MPS) is a provider of professional indemnity and advice to doctors, dentists and health professionals around the world. It is a mutual, not-for-profit organisation that offers its members (who number more than 265 000) help with legal and ethical problems that arise from their professional practice. These include clinical negligence claims, complaints, medical council inquiries, legal and ethical dilemmas, disciplinary procedures, inquests and fatal-accident inquiries.

The MPS medico-legal advisers manage a substantial and varied caseload. The telephone advisory service fields more than 18 000 calls a year. This places the MPS and the other medical defence organisations (MDOs) in a unique position, as they are able to hear directly from practising clinicians how they are affected by allegations and subsequent investigations.

Scope

The doctor–patient relationship requires boundaries to function effectively. These same boundaries may at times be crossed, broken or perceived to be crossed or broken, often leading to the breakdown of the relationship. The General Medical Council (GMC) comments:

Trust is a critical component in the doctor–patient partnership: patients must be able to trust doctors with their lives and health. In most successful doctor–patient relationships a professional boundary exists between doctor and patient. If this boundary is breached, this can undermine the patient's trust in their doctor, as well as the public's trust in the medical profession. (GMC, 2006).

Just as there are many different types of boundary, so there are as many ways for doctors to find themselves on the wrong side. Such transgressions can have significant consequences for the immediate therapeutic relationship and for the doctor's working life in general. The threat to the wider public confidence in the profession has resulted in regulatory bodies taking boundary infringements extremely seriously.

It is sexual boundaries that are thought of most often. Doctors who commit sexual crimes against their patients clearly raise concerns about public confidence in the profession and attract extensive media attention, but there are many more common transgressions, for instance treating a family member or taking part in an apparently consensual sexual relationship with a patient. The MPS regularly receives requests for assistance from doctors who have misused their position of trust to influence their patients' decisions on financial matters which favour the doctor: this can range from persuading patients to use pharmacies in which they have a financial interest to defrauding patients out of thousands of pounds.

It is commonly supposed that all the problems that end up with the regulators are a result of interactions with patients. However, regulatory bodies often review allegations of inappropriate behaviour involving staff members, or even situations arising in a doctor's personal life. The rationale is that such behaviour may represent 'moral turpitude' – that is, deficiencies in a person's moral standards – whether or not any patients are involved. Allegations or convictions for indecent assault, or those which involve offensive behaviour of a sexual or immoral nature, such as rape or pornography (especially child pornography), are viewed seriously and inevitably attract action against a doctor's registration.

Doctors also find themselves being brought to account for offences of much lesser magnitude. Some may question what relevance minor infractions could possibly have to the ability to practise medicine, and ask why a doctor is not entitled to a private life like anyone else in society. Such views are understandable, but regulatory bodies exist to protect the public and, in doing this, expect certain values and standards of personal behaviour. Appropriate behaviours are considered a prerequisite for the relationship

165

of trust and confidence that needs to exist between any healthcare provider and a patient.

Modern communication

The internet, email and social networking have changed many interactions recently. These informal media, with new rules of social interaction, have led doctors to find themselves both more readily accessible and less aware of the usual signs that they could pick up with face-to-face contact. The informality has led some doctors to find that online interactions have taken them to the other side of a boundary that they did not perceive. The new assumptions and customs of the virtual world will not apply when a doctor is being judged by a regulator. These media have also brought what previously might have been behaviour confined to a living room to a public audience. Employers and regulators may take a disapproving interest in the photos or videos that are posted on Facebook or YouTube.

The MPS experience

While there are insufficient data to be specific about the outcome of allegations of boundary violations, the MPS advisory service has assisted many doctors who have been accused of a boundary violation, including sexual misconduct. The overall impression is that the majority of these investigations result in the allegations being unproven. All cases opened with the MPS are allocated a short narrative 'headline', which it is possible to search for relevant terms. A search was carried out using a set of terms designed to identify as many cases as possible that might involve sexual misconduct. Searching all headlines of cases opened over 10 years (1 January 1999 to 31 December 2008) returned 545 cases. On reading the full headlines, 77 cases were excluded, as it was clear that they were not cases where the member of the MPS was accused of misconduct but were where the member sought advice on handling situations related to the sexual misconduct of others, such as providing a report to police in rape cases. This left 468 relevant cases (Table 14.1).

Table 14.1 Specialty of doctors accused of sexual boundary violations in the MPS case file, 1999–2008

Specialty	No. of cases	% of cases	% of membership
General practitioners	283	60.5	31.2
Psychiatrists	29	6.2	6.5
Gynaecologists	19	4.1	2.5
Accident and emergency specialists	17	3.6	2.2
Orthopaedic surgeons	16	3.4	2.7
Other	104	22.2	54.9

While some cases which involved allegations of boundary violations will not have been captured by the search terms, there is no reason to assume this should alter the patterns observed. The specialties traditionally assumed to be at a higher risk of allegations of sexual misconduct (general practice, psychiatry and gynaecology) do seem to have contacted the MPS more often for assistance with these types of allegation, but only general practitioners (GPs) were significantly overrepresented in terms of the proportion of the membership.

The data did not allow for analysis of the care environment – that is, National Health Service (NHS) or private practice. It was also not possible to differentiate between male and female doctors. In addition, these headlines were generated at the very beginning of the case and could not be used to see whether the allegations were ever substantiated.

Double jeopardy and beyond

Doctors, like other citizens, are expected to abide by the law of the jurisdiction they practise within but are also held to higher standards by their regulators. As a result, allegations can be brought in a number of different arenas, as illustrated in Box 14.2. The most serious allegations may attract criminal investigation and prosecution, but doctors have many other layers of regulation to work within, including the GMC standards of Good Medical Practice, employer disciplinary procedures and the NHS complaints procedure.

Doctors may find that they are subject to several parallel investigations in some or all of these areas. Each of the procedures differs in the form of investigation and the standard of proof required for doctors to have allegations found proven against them. This potentially leaves doctors in the position of having to defend themselves on the same allegations to several different tribunals, a situation often perceived as unfair and confusing.

Legal framework

In order to carry out their work, doctors often need to touch another person. This intrusion of bodily security is prevented from being a trespass only by the informed consent of a patient with capacity, without undue influence and with the presence of a legitimate medical reason. Otherwise this trespass would be actionable as a battery both in the criminal law and in the civil law of tort. Doctors who are accused of boundary violations are often unable to prove that there was valid consent and may be accused of having unduly influenced the patient or not having had a legitimate medical aim. It is thus the area of communication around consent that leads to many of the allegations doctors face.

Box 14.1 Multiple jeopardy illustrated: fictional case example

A 52-year-old GP principal in a five-partner practice saw a 16-year-old female with abdominal pain. The notes read: '16 F presents with 2/7 onset of lower abdominal pain, heaviness when voiding, no dysuria, no N&V, no change in bowel habit. Sexually active, using condoms, LMP 1/52 ago, not associated with intercourse. O/E Abdomen soft, mild tenderness suprapubicly, no peritonism. No masses. TUT +ve nitrates and Luc. 3/7 Trimethoprim. Return if persists or worsens.'

The following day the primary care trust (PCT) received a complaint from the mother of the patient saying that the doctor had done a 'personal examination' without consent or a chaperone and accusing the doctor of sexual assault: 'the doctor put his hand inside [her] daughter's pants and touched her private bits'. The practice was contacted by the police for a copy of the records and informed that the patient had made an allegation of sexual assault. The same day the doctor was contacted by the PCT and asked to stay away voluntarily from the practice pending a suspension hearing. Two days later the PCT suspended the doctor from its performers list, pending the police investigation. The fact of the doctor's suspension was reported in the local newspaper with the headline 'GP suspended over allegations of touching up teenage girl'.

The PCT reported the suspension to the GMC, which opened an investigation and invited the doctor to appear in front of the Interim Orders Panel (IOP). The IOP was held 10 days later (16 days after the consultation). The Panel determined that, owing to the nature of the allegation, it was necessary to place an order of suspension on the doctor's registration for 18 months in order to protect the public and in the wider public interest. This was again publicised in the local paper.

The partners in the practice decided that, owing to the adverse publicity, it was necessary to dissolve the partnership, which they were able to effect according to their partnership agreement without providing reasons. The debt in the practice was deemed to be equivalent to the value of the practice, so the doctor received no monies. The partnership then re-formed with the four remaining partners.

The doctor's teenage daughters received anonymous notes and text messages at school saying 'What is it like to live with Dr Perv?' The eldest daughter felt unable to attend school.

The police interviewed the patient formally on the day of the IOP. The patient described the doctor examining her abdomen, asking her to undo her trousers so that he could feel all of her tummy and described the doctor feeling so far down he reached her pubic bone. She did not think anything was wrong at the time until she discussed it with her mother who 'went mad'. The police determined that no criminal action had occurred and closed their case without interviewing the doctor.

The PCT decided it was necessary to investigate the doctor, concentrating on the consent process and any potential breach of the PCT's chaperone policy. They interviewed the patient, her mother, members of the practice and then the doctor. The PCT decided to lift the suspension and forwarded the result of their investigation to the GMC.

The IOP reviewed the suspension at 6 months and decided to lift it. The GMC wrote to the doctor saying that its decision was that 'there was insufficient evidence to establish your fitness to practice may be impaired' and therefore 'no further action will be taken'.

The doctor was unable to find work within the same town and ended up working 75 miles away. This was followed by marital discord and eventual separation. The doctor's eldest daughter struggled with her A-levels owing to the stress at home and failed to achieve her expected grades, thereby failing to get her place at medical school.

The Sexual Offences Act 2003 introduced a revised legislative framework for the definition and prosecution of sexual offences. It is important to realise that the same common-law principles discussed above with regard to consent will apply when interpreting the Sexual Offences Act (see Box 14.2). For example, the administration of a sedative could be classified as administering a substance with intent (defined in Box 14.2), even if the patient apparently consented to the administration for what was made out to be a legitimate aim but without knowing the actual aim of sexual gratification.

There was concern at first that these definitions would lead to an increase in the numbers of doctors facing criminal investigations, particularly with some of the lesser offences which previously were difficult to prosecute. However, the MPS has not noticed a significant increase in doctors seeking assistance with this sort of investigation and the number of such cases is very small.

Regulatory framework

GMC

In order to practise medicine, a doctor must maintain his or her position on the list of registered medical practitioners maintained by the GMC. Since medical practice is the sole source of income for nearly all doctors, the fear of losing registration is great and will be the primary concern once any threat of criminal prosecution is over. After a referral, the GMC begins its investigation by writing to all organisations to whom the practitioner offers medical services, even if only on a voluntary basis. The investigation proceeds until it is felt there is enough information to decide whether or not there is a realistic prospect of finding the doctor's fitness to practise to be impaired. If so, the GMC will move towards holding a 'fitness to practise' hearing. (The role of the GMC is considered at length in Chapter 16.)

The GMC may refer cases in which boundary violations are alleged to an interim orders panel (IOP). Although the resulting hearing is not public, the fact that a particular doctor is to appear and the order made are public. This adds to any media attention the case may already have, while the private nature of the proceedings can sometimes allow the press to speculate on the precise nature of the allegations. Although media attention cannot be prevented, MDOs representing doctors at such hearings will usually offer a media relations or press office service so that doctors can seek advice on what sort of comment to make and even how best to say 'no comment'. Press interest is often predictable, particularly in cases involving sexual misconduct or high-profile doctors, and pre-prepared statements can be made . It is often harder to influence more modern forms of reporting such as online forums or blogs. Information can be reported by untraceable sources, therefore making misreporting more common and unaccountable. MDOs assist in getting reports retracted or corrected when necessary.

Box 14.2 Definitions of terms used in the Sexual Offences Act 2003

Rape
Rape is now classified as penetration by the penis of somebody's vagina, anus or mouth, without their consent. Rape can be committed against men or women, but since it involves penile penetration it is committed only by men.

Assault by penetration
Under this new law, it is an offence to penetrate the anus or vagina of someone else with any part of the body or with an object, if the penetration is sexual and if the person does not consent.

Sexual assault
This law covers any kind of intentional sexual touching of somebody else without their consent. It includes touching any part of their body, clothed or unclothed, either with a part of the body or with an object.

Causing a person to engage in a sexual activity without consent
This law covers any kind of sexual activity without consent. For instance it would apply to a woman who forces a man to penetrate her, or an abuser who makes a victim engage in masturbation.

Administering a substance with intent
This new law makes it a separate offence to give someone any substance – for instance spiking their drink – without their consent, and with the intention of stupefying them so that sexual activity can take place. In this instance, sexual activity could include stripping or taking pornographic photographs of them. Someone can be charged with this offence in addition to any separate charge for rape or sexual assault. They can also be charged when the intended sexual activity did not take place, for instance when someone sees what is going on and intervenes to stop it.

Other 'intent' offences
Two new laws – 'committing an offence with intent' and 'trespass with intent' – cover situations where abusers commit one offence (such as violence, trespass, or detaining someone against their will) with the intention of then committing a sexual offence.

Other offences
Other offences under the Act include exposure (or 'flashing'), voyeurism, sex in public toilets, and sex with animals or with corpses. Voyeurism is a new offence which applies to watching people involved in private acts without their consent. It includes setting up, viewing or recording people through electronic equipment such as webcams or cameras.

Source: Home Office Communications Directorate (2004).

Performers list

The majority of career-grade doctors in the UK are GPs and face yet another level of regulation. Since the introduction of the National Health Service (Performers Lists) Regulations in 2004 all doctors wishing to offer primary care medical services to NHS patients must be on the 'performers list' of the primary care trust (PCT). This requires compliance with the 2004 Regulations, which provide for investigation of concerns – with the potential for suspension from the list pending the outcome of the investigation and hearings to decide whether to remove a performer from the list. Furthermore, a PCT can apply to the First-Tier Tribunal (Primary Health Lists) for a national disqualification, thereby preventing a doctor working as a GP in the NHS and essentially ending that doctor's career. It should be noted that this is carried out by PCTs, which are not expert regulators, even if they are experienced in the management of performers. When faced with the task of investigating and holding hearings into a doctor's conduct, they may have difficulties ensuring that their actions are perceived as fair.

NHS disciplinary action

For those doctors who are not GPs, and for some employed GPs, there is the prospect of facing disciplinary action governed by the Department of Health (2003) document *Maintaining High Professional Standards in the Modern NHS* (MHPS). This brings the discipline of doctors for conduct issues within the local procedures used to discipline any other employee. It also specifically deals with doctors who are accused of a criminal offence – which may be the case in allegations of serious boundary violations.

Allegations of serious boundary violations inevitably attract a discussion about exclusion during an ensuing investigation but some trusts are amen-able to the suggestion that any potential risk can be dealt with by alternative means. The MPS has been successful in returning some members to either restricted or supervised practice while the investigation is carried out.

The MHPS allows doctors to be accompanied at all stages of the process by a companion, who may be: another NHS employee; an official or lay representative of the British Medical Association, British Dental Association or defence organisation; or a friend, partner or spouse. The MHPS was thought to exclude the doctor from being accompanied by a lawyer. The phrase 'The companion may be legally qualified but he or she will not be acting in a legal capacity' has been a source of litigation and would seem to have been clarified as a result of a case supported by the MPS (*Kulkarni v. Milton Keynes Hospital NHS Foundation Trust*, [2009] EWCA Civ 789). Lady Justice Smith's view was that a denial of legal representation to a doctor who faced the possibility of dismissal would be a breach of article 6 of the European Convention on Human Rights (the right to a fair trial). In providing this opinion Lady Justice Smith stated:

the National Health Service is, to all intents and purposes, a single employer for the whole country. Indeed, for a trainee doctor, that is literally true as a doctor cannot complete his training in the private sector. If [a doctor in training] is found guilty on this charge he will be unemployable as a doctor and will never complete his training.

In recognising the NHS as a monopoly employer, she highlighted one of the major problems faced by doctors who are accused of boundary violations.

Alert notices

Finally, doctors or other health professionals who receive an adverse outcome at a disciplinary hearing for allegations associated with boundary violations are likely also to attract an 'alert notice' or letter. These notices are issued by the strategic health authority (SHA) and currently take the form of a letter which is distributed to specific NHS bodies requesting that if the subject of the alert notice seeks employment they should seek a written reference from a named person within the original organisation.

Where do doctors get help?

While all of the UK's MDOs will in some way assist doctors facing these sorts of allegation, their arrangements differ. Doctors who are the subject of allegations of sexual misconduct may seek assistance from the MPS, which is a mutual society offering discretionary indemnity to its members. In practice, the MPS would normally assist members with allegations that arise out of their professional practice in whatever forum they are brought. The MPS would also usually assist members with investigations and proceedings that are brought by the GMC irrespective of what part of the doctor's life was involved.

Doctors may also seek assistance with allegations from their trade union organisations, such as the British Medical Association and the Hospital Consultants and Specialists Association. This is of particular relevance to allegations arising out of personal conduct that attracts disciplinary action by a doctor's employer.

Advice

The MPS is often approached for advice on avoiding allegations of sexual misconduct and has offered guidance to medical professionals in this area over the years. Comprehensive guidance has also been provided by the GMC (*Maintaining Boundaries*; General Medical Council, 2006) and by the Council for Healthcare Regulatory Excellence (2008). These publications have been welcomed by healthcare professionals and their advisers. Both documents place an emphasis on clear and effective communication, thereby recognising that complaints of inappropriate behaviour frequently arise from misunderstanding, rather than wilful wrongdoing (see Box 14.3).

Intimate examinations

Doctors regularly find themselves working in close physical proximity to patients, which creates a need to be mindful of how their actions may

---

Box 14.3 Clear and effective communication

Clear communication with patients helps to avoid misunderstandings. During diagnosis or treatment healthcare professionals should explain what they are going to do and why. They must communicate this in a way that the patient can understand and that takes into account the patient's particular communication requirements. In particular, a healthcare professional should:

- explain why certain questions need to be asked
- explain why any examination or procedure is necessary
- explain what will happen during any examination or procedure and ensure the patient has understood
- find out what the patient wants to know about their condition and its treatment
- give the patient an opportunity to ask questions
- if necessary, use an appropriate interpreter
- obtain the patient's permission before the assessment or treatment and record that permission has been obtained
- make sure patients know that they can communicate any discomfort or concern and that they can stop an examination or procedure at any time.

Source: Council for Healthcare Regulatory Excellence (2008).

---

be perceived or interpreted, however innocent or well intentioned. The physical examination is a time when clear boundaries are of the utmost importance. Many of the allegations have arisen in connection with an intimate examination or one that the patient or relative interpreted as intimate.

It is important to recognise that an intimate examination may be an everyday occurrence for a doctor but unfamiliar to the patient. This is particularly important in specialties where intimate examinations are routine, such as gynaecology. The doctor, who is familiar with carrying out physical examinations, may have a different concept of 'intimate' from the patient; additionally, different patients will have different ideas.

The GMC is sensitive to this point:

Whenever you examine a patient you should be sensitive to what they may perceive as intimate. This is likely to include examinations of breasts, genitalia and rectum, but could also include any examination where it is necessary to touch or even be close to the patient. (General Medical Council, 2006, para. 9)

This again highlights the importance of communication when attempting to avoid difficulties associated with intimate examination (see also Chapter 10).

Chaperones

Despite publishing articles on the sensible use of chaperones, and advising in lectures and individually, the MPS continues to see cases which might have been avoided if this issue had been dealt with appropriately. There is a consensus that, wherever possible, patients should be offered the choice of having an impartial observer, or chaperone, present during an examination that the patient considers to be intimate. The issues raised are often associated with the choice of chaperone and what to do if there is no one available or the patient declines the offer.

Discussion about chaperones should be recorded in the medical records whether the result is that a chaperone is present or not. The GMC (2006, para. 13) recommends:

You should record any discussion about chaperones and its outcome. If a chaperone is present, you should record that fact and make a note of their identity. If the patient does not want a chaperone, you should record that the offer was made and declined.

Many incidents could have been eased if the doctor had offered a chaperone and made good notes of the discussion.

A chaperone should ideally be a healthcare professional trained in what is required, though there may be situations where a relative or friend is appropriate. Many primary care organisations also train non-healthcare professionals in order that they can assist. The GMC (2006, para. 11) lists the properties of an ideal chaperone:

- sensitive, and respectful of the patient's dignity and confidentiality
- prepared to reassure the patient if they show signs of distress or discomfort
- familiar with the procedures involved in routine intimate examination
- prepared to raise concerns about a doctor if misconduct occurs.

Sometimes it will not be possible to find a suitably trained chaperone or one with whom both the patient and the doctor are comfortable. Such situations should be avoided where possible but the doctor must prioritise the patient's needs and there will be situations where it is essential to continue. In most cases, though, the sensible approach is to offer the patient an alternative time or place for the examination to be carried out, when a chaperone who is acceptable to both patient and doctor is available. The doctor, of course, must first consider the effects such a delay might have on the patient's health.

No arrangement provides absolute protection against allegations that inappropriate things were said or done. Such allegations have, in the past, related to acts which are said to have occurred when:

- a nurse/assistant leaves the room, even briefly
- a nurse/assistant has turned around or is occupied with other activities
- the third party happens not to be observing what is happening.

Warning signs

Many doctors have said after the event that there had been warning signs that a doctor–patient relationship was heading in the wrong direction and if these had been spotted the breach of the boundary or the allegation of the breach might have been avoided (see Council for Healthcare Regulatory Excellence, 2008, p. 4).

Patient behaviour

Patients may directly inform doctors of their attraction towards them or may exhibit more subtle signs, such as refusing to see any other doctor, or making excuses to run into them both in the place of practice and outside.

Doctors' behaviour

It is important that all doctors are aware of behaviours which, while not constituting a breach of boundaries, may be warning signs. Some examples of these behaviours are:

- frequently thinking about the patient on a personal level
- looking forward to seeing the patient with a sense of anticipation
- allowing consultations to run over time, even though there is no clinical reason for it
- giving the patient preferential treatment – for example cutting another patient's consultation short to make room for the patient or expediting a referral for non-clinical reasons
- treating the patient as 'special' – for example showing unusual deference, 'going the extra mile'
- divulging personal information
- creating opportunities to see the patient.

Dealing with warning signs

If doctors are concerned that a patient may be attracted to them to a level that may interfere with the professional relationship, or find themselves attracted to a patient, the most important piece of advice is to seek advice. A doctor in this situation should discuss concerns with a colleague or could seek advice from the MDO.

It may be possible to create a professional environment again that allows for an effective therapeutic relationship to continue. This will usually require the doctor to be clear to the patient where the boundaries lie and what sort of behaviours are unacceptable. This sort of intervention must be carried out early in the process to be successful.

There are situations where the continuation of the professional relationship is not possible. The doctor is responsible for ensuring that alternative arrangements for care of the patient are made and that such arrangements are made in a way that does not compromise care or leave the patient feeling he or she has done anything wrong. It is again advisable that the doctor seeks advice when making these arrangements.

Conclusion

Doctors may be subject to allegations about boundary violations in a number of different areas. The experience is always very stressful and is a direct threat to a doctor's livelihood. MDOs can provide assistance and advice throughout and can advise on how best to avoid the possibility of such complaints arising.

References

Council for Healthcare Regulatory Excellence (2008) *Clear Sexual Boundaries Between Healthcare Professionals and Patients: Responsibilities of Healthcare Professionals*. CHRE. Available online at http://www.chre.org.uk/_img/pics/library/0801_Clear_Sexual_boundaries_professionals.pdf.

Department of Health (2003) *Maintaining High Professional Standards in the Modern NHS: A Framework for the Initial Handling of Concerns about Doctors and Dentists in the NHS*. Available online at http://www.dh.gov.uk/en/Publicationsandstatistics/Publications/PublicationsPolicyAndGuidance/DH_4080677 (accessed June 2010).

General Medical Council (2006) *Supplementary Guidance: Maintaining Boundaries*. GMC. Available online at http://www.gmc-uk.org/static/documents/content/Maintaining_Boundaries.pdf (accessed June 2010).

Home Office Communications Directorate (2004) *Adults: Safer from Sexual Crime. The Sexual Offences Act 2003*. Home Office.

Kulkarni v. Milton Keynes Hospital NHS Foundation Trust, [2009] EWCA Civ 789.

CHAPTER 15

Regulation and its capacity to minimise abuse by professionals

Julie Stone

Overview

Evidence from complaints and cases concerning fitness to practise reveals that professional abuse occurs across the range of regulated health professions. While regulation may not be able to prevent determined sexual predators from offending, coordinated processes could do much to reduce the risk to patients. The failure of government and regulators to implement comprehensive strategies relating to sexual boundaries constitutes a regulatory failure. Drawing on work undertaken by the Council for Healthcare Regulatory Excellence's 'Clear Sexual Boundaries' project, the chapter looks at some of the areas where regulation has been strengthened in relation to boundaries and what more needs to be done.

Background

As detailed elsewhere in this volume, in recent years there have been several highly publicised inquiries into cases of abuse perpetrated by health professionals (see, for example, Box 6.1, p. 65, on Michael Haslam; Box 6.2, p. 66, on William Kerr; Box 10.1, p. 115, on Clifford Ayling; and Box 11.1, p. 131, on David Britten). Each case involved serious sexual abuse of multiple patients over extended periods and the inquiries highlighted how opportunities to detect problems had been missed. Boundary transgressions are of concern to regulators, both in respect of the severity of harm caused to the individuals who are abused, and to the extent that the media reporting such cases of abuse diminishes trust and confidence in the health professions.

In 2006, in response to the Ayling and Kerr/Haslam Inquiries, the Department of Health commissioned the Council for Healthcare Regulatory Excellence (CHRE) to undertake a programme of regulatory research aimed at protecting patients by minimising the likelihood of boundary violations. Recognising boundary issues to be a significant patient safety issue, the

CHRE had already initiated an internal programme of work in this area, commissioning POPAN (the Prevention Of Professional Abuse Network, later Witness) to compare the guidance on this issue produced by all of the UK healthcare regulators (Coe *et al*, 2005). That research highlighted significant discrepancies between them. The CHRE work included a review and analysis of the literature on boundary violations (Halter *et al*, 2007), and the production of guidelines for professionals, patients, educators, and fitness-to-practise panels dealing with boundary allegations (Council for Healthcare Regulatory Excellence, 2008*a*–*c*). In keeping with its statutory remit, the CHRE's guidance was targeted primarily at the statutorily regulated healthcare professions, although psychotherapists and other non-regulated professions were also represented throughout the project.

The lack of systematic data collection in the UK makes it hard to detect the prevalence of boundary violations with accuracy (see Chapter 5). However, proxy markers, including complaints and fitness-to-practise findings, indicate that boundary concerns are not uncommon among regulated health professions. *Safeguarding Patients* (Department of Health, 2007*a*) states that very broad-brush estimates in other countries suggest that the prevalence could be as high as 6–7% of health professionals, drawing on research provided to the CHRE (Coe *et al*, 2005). According to the CHRE, one health professional a week is struck off by regulators for sexual misconduct. Since 2005, over 250 cases of sexual misconduct have been considered by health professional regulators (Council for Healthcare Regulatory Excellence, 2009). As there is every reason to suspect high levels of underreporting of abuse, this is an alarming statistic, especially as most regulators now have guidance prohibiting inappropriate behaviour.

Given that issuing guidance on sexual boundaries has been the main regulatory response to the inquiries and the CHRE's 'Clear Sexual Boundaries' project, it begs the question of how far guidelines, in isolation, prevent boundary violations. The purpose of this chapter, therefore, is to explore what else regulators need to do as part of a comprehensive strategy to minimise abuse. Regulators cannot achieve this single-handedly, and reducing risk will require them to work in concert with registrants, higher-education institutions (HEIs) and employers to ensure a culture of zero tolerance towards the abuse of vulnerable patients, defined in statute to include adults receiving any form of healthcare.

Potential areas of regulatory interface

The overriding function of professional regulation is to protect the public. There are currently nine healthcare regulators in the UK: the General Chiropractic Council, General Dental Council, General Medical Council, General Optical Council, General Osteopathic Council, Health Professions Council, Nursing and Midwifery Council, Pharmaceutical Society of

Northern Ireland, and the General Pharmaceutical Council. Each regulator has four key statutory responsibilities. These are:

1   setting standards for pre-registration education and training
2   maintaining a register of professionals
3   disseminating codes of ethics/standards of practice
4   operating fitness-to-practise processes.

Each element has a potential role in minimising boundary abuses. Abuse can be minimised overtly and more subtly, and it is important that regulators consider the totality of their regulatory processes. Registration, for example, can ensure that a person with a criminal conviction for a sexual offence is not admitted to a professional register. But registrars can also ensure that the language tests they impose on non-UK/non-European Union applicants require applicants to demonstrate sufficient communication skills to be able to forge good and safe therapeutic relationships. Similarly, fitness-to-practise processes can erase ('strike off') or suspend a practitioner who has breached sexual boundaries, or impose conditions to ensure that an offending practitioner is prevented from direct patient contact. Less directly, the provision by a regulator of advocacy support could help someone to initiate a fitness-to-practise allegation who might otherwise lack the confidence to do so.

Education and training

Whereas fitness to practise is the most visible aspect of the regulatory process, the area of regulation most likely to prevent practitioners from offending is education and training. Healthcare practitioners enjoy a significant degree of autonomy and freedom in how they carry out their role, and much healthcare practice takes place in unsupervised settings. This means that the onus on protecting patients rests primarily with individual practitioners, working with integrity and within their codes of practice. Effective education and training should cultivate the knowledge, skills and attitudes which underpin ethical practice, and ensure that those entering clinical practice appreciate the ethical and legal requirements of their role, including the duty to create and maintain safe boundaries.

Pre-registration education, outcomes and competencies

While regulators tend not to impose a core curriculum, they do set out benchmark statements indicating the outcomes a course needs to deliver, and scope-of-practice requirements, which highlight the competencies a registrant will be expected to have in order to join a professional register. These inform the course content delivered by HEIs, whose courses are approved by the regulator as recognised qualifications for the purposes of registration. Accordingly, regulators can ensure that students acquire competencies to maintain safe boundaries, such as effective communication skills, appropriate history-taking skills, and knowledge about safeguarding policies and working with vulnerable groups.

Where, when and what to teach

Professionals who have received education and training about boundaries may be less likely to offend (Halter *et al*, 2007). Additionally, education and training can highlight the professional responsibility of colleagues to speak out if they suspect abuse or poor performance on the part of colleagues. Little is known about what sorts of boundaries training are most likely to minimise abuse, or when this learning should take place, and this would be useful research for the regulators or the CHRE to commission. Work to date recommends that concepts such as relationships of trust, imbalance of power and patients' best interests should be an integral part of boundaries training and that this subject could be incorporated into ethics and law courses, personal and professional development and clinical skills training (Council for Healthcare Regulatory Excellence, 2008*a*). As much healthcare delivery is now provided by teams, training about boundaries could also be incorporated as part of multidisciplinary team learning, especially as professionals have a duty to report colleagues' misconduct or poor perfor- mance, and inquiries have flagged up the difficulty of reporting more senior colleagues. Of course, it is not just what students learn but also what they see that shapes their development, and positive role modelling is another way that students learn how to treat patients with dignity and respect.

The CHRE's 2008 report on learning about sexual boundaries highlighted the need for boundary issues to be taught as a *mainstream issue*, and not something which applies only to an aberrant few (Council for Healthcare Regulatory Excellence, 2008*a*). Boundary maintenance is more than the avoidance of inappropriate sexual relationships. All healthcare practitioners need to be aware that they may be vulnerable to breaching boundaries in certain situations. Learning about boundaries in a supportive, non-judgemental way protects practitioners as well as patients, by acknowledging sexualised feelings but teaching students how to protect themselves and patients. Education must also equip practitioners to recognise patients who have poor sense of boundaries, and knowing how to deflect inappropriate behaviours of patients and keep them safe.

Continuing professional development, revalidation and post-registration education and training

Pre-registration education is not the only point at which boundary issues can or should be taught; arguably, registrants may be more responsive to learning about boundaries later on in their careers. Nonetheless, as many healthcare students have clinical placements from early on in their courses, they need to know the basic principles around patient safety, consent to treatment and working with vulnerable groups. Although regulators are concerned primarily with the pre-registration curriculum, they also have a statutory role in ensuring that practitioners remain fit to practise. This is currently achieved by requiring registrants to undertake continuing professional development (CPD) in order to remain registered. Notwithstanding the self-directed nature of CPD, some regulators specify mandatory components of it. Given the large numbers of registrants who have never received any training on boundaries, this could be a way to improve public protection. Regulators may also consider accrediting CPD courses, to ensure the quality of teaching and learning about boundaries.

Within medicine, the bulk of post-registration learning is orchestrated by the medical Royal Colleges. Several of the Royal Colleges participated in the CHRE's 'Clear Sexual Boundaries' project, and used the CHRE's guidelines as an impetus to develop their own, profession-specific guidance. The Royal College of Psychiatrists, for example, has issued explicit guidelines in relation to sexual boundaries in psychiatry (Royal College of Psychiatrists, 2007). Regulators need to work closely with Royal Colleges and post-registration trainers to ensure that there is an appropriate level of training in this area. Developments in relation to revalidation, set out in the government's white paper *Trust, Assurance and Safety* (Department of Health, 2007*b*), might provide a further opportunity to ensure that practitioners have undertaken training on boundaries.

Registration

The main hallmark of a statutorily regulated profession is the maintenance of a register of appropriately qualified professionals. Use of a professional title, such as 'osteopath' or 'midwife', is protected by law, and it is a criminal offence for people to use a protected title or to hold themselves out as registered professionals if they are not on the register. In a statutory environment, being 'struck off' effectively prohibits a practitioner from practising in the field.

Admittance to the register: good health and character and absence of convictions

In order to gain admittance onto a professional register, applicants must possess a recognised qualification, and must also satisfy the regulator that they are of 'good character'. Although 'good character' requirements vary from regulator to regulator, most require a combination of a declaration of good health from the applicant's doctor, a sign-off letter from the HEI awarding the registering qualification, and an absence of criminal convictions. Each provides a somewhat limited safeguard against future boundary abuses. The sign-off letter from an HEI is more or less automatic, although there is greater scope for flagging up future problems now that some HEIs have introduced student fitness-to-practise procedures. A criminal conviction for a sexual offence would almost certainly disbar someone from registration, but, of course, not all offenders will have been prosecuted or convicted for previous offences. Currently, a check with the Criminal Records Bureau (CRB) is required of new registrants.

The process of registration offers some reassurance to patients that professionals who are on the register do not have criminal convictions, have been trained to the standards required of the profession, adhere to a code of ethics, and are subject to fitness-to-practise proceedings. But registration provides only partial protection. Given the number of boundary cases which come before regulators' fitness-to-practise panels, and the fact that all of the inquiries have involved statutorily regulated health professionals, registration of professionals can be only part of a coordinated strategy to minimise abuse.

Making the register accessible

Outside formal healthcare environments such as hospitals or clinics, it will not always be obvious to a patient who is, and who is not, a statutorily regulated professional. Part of good regulation must be helping patients to protect themselves, by making it easy for them to check the register, and by giving them accessible information to empower them to express concerns if they do not feel that behaviour or conduct is appropriate. This may require regulators and employers to provide advocacy support for patients so that they can be supported through the process of raising a complaint.

Acting on reciprocal findings

Another important registration safeguard would be the ability of regulators to take into account fitness-to-practise findings from other regulatory bodies, whether in the UK or elsewhere. This is particularly important in relation to registrants from the European Union (EU), given their freedom of movement. Whereas provisions are improving within the EU as a result of the Healthcare Professionals Crossing Borders initiative, reciprocal arrangements outside the EU are less robust. Reciprocal arrangements would prohibit someone who had been struck off one register for sexual misconduct applying to join another professional regulator.

Regulators should also be able to take account of findings from non-statutorily regulated professions and vice versa in relation to registration and fitness to practise. People who have been struck off any healthcare register should not be working in a position of trust with patients or vulnerable groups. The problem currently is that someone who has been

---

Box 15.1 Working privately after having been struck off

In a recent case, an arts therapist struck off the Health Professions Council's register for impaired fitness to practise remains able to continue to work as a private therapist because of the current lack of statutory regulation of counselling and psychotherapy. Proven allegations included the therapist falling asleep and sending text messages during therapy sessions, insulting a client by swearing at her, taking a holiday with a client, allowing clients to provide him with business services free of charge, and smoking cannabis in front of clients. The Health Professions Council's panel found that the therapist did not have regard to the need for clear and consistent boundaries, or to the extreme caution that would be required if a generally accepted boundary were to be crossed, and found him to have a cavalier attitude towards the needs of clients and the requirement to follow clear guidelines.

Source: http://www.hpc-uk.org/complaints/hearings/index.asp?id=981

---

erased from a statutory register may simply continue to work, for example as an unregulated counsellor or psychotherapist, which is one reason why statutory regulation is so important (Box 15.1).

Interface with employers

The registrar (usually the regulator's chief executive) is not the only person with responsibilities in this regard. Safeguards need to be reinforced by employers, who play a vital role in ensuring that references are taken up, induction training is given to all staff, and employers are familiar with employment codes and local reporting mechanisms. Specific advice has been disseminated to employers in this regard (NHS Employers, 2008). In order to help employers fulfil their functions, regulators should ensure that the professional register is accessible and up to date. Consideration is currently being given to the regulator's register being the portal where all concerns about a registrant could be detailed, although this will require legislative amendment to take effect.

Professional guidelines and codes of ethics

The main responsibility for acting ethically rests with the individual practitioner. In the context of safe boundaries, this means attracting into health professions individuals with high levels of personal integrity, and ensuring that education, training and CPD equip them to deal with the challenging boundary issues they are likely to face in practice. Superficially, it would be comforting to think that as long as regulators prohibited unethical behaviour in their codes, all practitioners would act appropriately. In reality, this is not the case, as witnessed by the volume of fitness-to-practise cases which regulators have to consider each year. Nonetheless, research has shown that greater awareness of professional guidelines and sanctions is associated with reduced prevalence (Halter *et al*, 2007). Accordingly, this section will consider the extent to which codes have a role in minimising the risk of abuse.

Functions of codes

Regulators set out their expectations of practitioners in their codes of ethics, and registered professionals agree to be bound by these codes. The dissemination of codes is a statutory responsibility, serving at least four distinct functions:

- to set out the values which underpin a profession and the responsibilities of practitioners, so that they know what is expected of them
- to ensure that members of the public know what is required of practitioners so that they can hold them to account
- to sets out a baseline of what is required of practitioners, which is capable of being used in fitness-to-practise hearings, employment disciplinary cases, complaints or court cases
- to help change organisational cultures by making it a specific requirement for registered professionals to report poor practice or misconduct of colleagues.

Codes of ethics try to reconcile two distinct tasks – articulating the values and principles which underpin the profession, and setting out a list of prohibited activities. This results in some codes sounding a positive, advisory tone, while others read as a long list of prohibited activities. Specifically, there has been a long-standing prohibition in most codes of entering into sexual relationships with patients, and few practitioners can be unaware that they should not have sex with their patients. However, boundary issues are far broader than prohibiting sexual relationships with patients and codes need to reflect the whole spectrum of behaviours and activities which are characterised by abuse of power relationships. This is likely to follow from an understanding of the values underpinning healthcare, such as the need to respect patient autonomy, the need to promote patients' interests and the need to protect them from harm.

Specific boundaries guidance

Although regulators have always prohibited sex with patients, they have varied in the amount of guidance they provide around boundaries. A study commissioned by the CHRE found that each of the regulators issued its own guidelines on boundaries. Accordingly, as one of its work-streams, the CHRE was commissioned to develop template guidelines for healthcare professionals on sexual boundaries, either as stand-alone guidelines or as a basis for profession-specific advice (Council for Healthcare Regulatory Excellence, 2008d). Several of the regulators have now issued discrete, boundary-specific guidance for their registrants to supplement prohibitions in their generic codes of ethics, including the Nursing and Midwifery Council (2009), the Royal Pharmaceutical Society of Great Britain (2008) and the General Medical Council (2006).

Ex-patients, dual relationships and self-disclosure

Despite the availability of guidelines, practitioners remain confused about certain key issues. Three recur frequently:

1   Who is an 'ex-patient' and when, if ever, is it appropriate to have a sexual or social relationship with ex-patients?
2   When, if ever, are dual relationships appropriate (e.g. treating friends, colleagues or family members)?
3   What level of self-disclosure (of the professional's personal informa-tion) is permissible?

These uncertainties reflect the difficulties in making absolute rules about this aspect of the therapeutic relationship. In the case of relationships with ex-patients, there are sound reasons for prohibiting relationships with anyone who is, or has ever been, a patient, based on their ongoing vulnerability, and the initial power imbalance in the relationship. But the other two areas of confusion, around dual relationships and self-disclosure, highlight that codes of practice are not a substitute for the exercise of professional judgement. While dual relationships may be generally inadvisable, in certain situations they may be unavoidable, particularly for practitioners working in rural settings, or in client-led services. Dual relationships require skilful and subtle negotiation, with a focus on the client's best interests, as opposed to an absolute prohibition. Similarly, self-disclosure may be an indication that a practitioner is using the professional relationship for his or her own ends, or it may indicate a therapeutically justified strategy to demonstrate empathy and increase the patient's trust. Again, this will depend on the individual patient's best interests. This highlights that while codes can give general advice, they are not a substitute for the practitioner making ethical decisions on the basis of all of the facts of the case.

Enhancing the deterrent effect of codes

Another consideration is the extent to which codes of ethics act as a deter-rent. Put bluntly, codes of ethics do not, of themselves, stop misconduct. There may be very little a regulator can do to deter a determined sexual predator, just as no code of ethics would have prevented Harold Shipman from mass murder. But what codes can do is to send out a strong statement about the sorts of behaviour that professions will not tolerate, and to support a strong organisational culture prohibiting abuse.

Codes can be made more meaningful when they are highly publicised and visible, kept regularly up to date, informed by fitness-to-practise cases, and reviewed regularly. Rather than trying to capture every possible prohibited boundary behaviour, registrants may find it more illustrative to see examples of what sorts of issues have resulted in adverse fitness-to-practise findings. Specifically, regulators might also consider posting research articles and anonymised victim impact statements on their websites to inform practitioners about why boundary breaches are so destructive.

Fitness to practise

As the most publicly visible aspect of regulatory control, fitness-to-practise adjudications have both a deterrent and a declaratory role. (The General Medical Council's function here is detailed in Chapter 16.) Exercising the right to strike a practitioner off the register stops that individual from harming patients in a professional capacity, and sends out a strong message that a regulator will deal robustly with violations of trust. Effective regulation uses information from fitness-to-practise cases to inform its other work, for example disseminating guidance on areas which give rise to repeated complaints, and ensuring that these issues are fed into the pre-registration curriculum. However, fitness to practise is, by its very nature, retrospective and, like criminal prosecution, comes into play only after harm has already occurred. In common with criminal prosecutions, fitness to practise requires a patient (or family member) to come forward and make a complaint. Patients who have been abused may not feel able to make a complaint to a regulator. Evidence to the Kerr/Haslam Inquiry revealed that even where patients had complained, they were not always believed. How might fitness-to-practise mechanisms be strengthened to minimise abuse in the future?

Consistency of approach and consistency of outcome

Regulators need to send out strong and consistent messages about practitioners who abuse. Most regulators have adopted indicative sanctions, which indicate the appropriate regulatory response when allegations have been proven in particular areas. Serious boundary failures will ordinarily result in erasure (being 'struck off') or, at the very least, a period of suspension if there is extremely persuasive mitigation. Problems, in terms of public protection and public reassurance, arise when fitness-to-practise panels impose lenient penalties which are inconsistent with the regulator's own indicative sanctions, for example only imposing conditions on a general practitioner who entered into a sexual relationship with a vulnerable female patient. In such cases the CHRE can refer a final decision of a fitness-to-practise panel to the High Court in cases of 'undue leniency' under section 29 of the National Health Service Reform and Health Care Professions Act 2002; nonetheless, regulators should ensure that panel members are adequately trained and are familiar with indicative sanctions and the outcome of CHRE appeals. The CHRE has recently undertaken a project to look at whether a common approach to sanctions across the nine regulators could be adopted (Council for Healthcare Regulatory Excellence, 2008*d*). A coherent and robust approach would be helpful in this area, as there can be little justification for a differential approach to boundary violations across the regulated professions.

The development of rehabilitation packages

The UK has been slow in developing rehabilitation packages for healthcare professionals who have been found guilty of more minor breaches of sexual boundaries, or as a precursor to readmission to the register after a period of suspension. While regulators have imposed *ad hoc* conditions, there has been little systematic work to develop programmes to prevent reoffending by healthcare practitioners, or to develop criteria for determining who might respond to such rehabilitation (leaving aside policy issues of how far the public would support retraining of 'offending' practitioners). This contrasts with the USA, where rehabilitation packages have been available for many years (see Chapter 13 on remediation). Failure to have access to such programmes means that the options for professionals who might be rehabilitated consist only of striking them off, or suspending them, either of which may be overly cautious from the professional perspective, or giving a warning, which may be an inadequate safeguard. Rehabilitation packages usually require extensive psychological screening, to flag up practitioners with pathological issues around boundaries which might require treatment and support. This is an important area for regulatory research and development.

The conduct of fitness-to-practise hearings

How a regulator organises and conducts its fitness-to-practise process will have a bearing on the outcome for all parties involved. A badly handled hearing can cause further harm and suffering to a complainant. With obvious parallels to rape prosecutions, loss of confidence in the system may deter others from coming forward. By contrast, hearings that are both safe for complainants and well thought through will both be fair and inspire public confidence. Recommendations for good practice were set out in the document *Clear Sexual Boundaries Between Healthcare Professionals and Patients: Guidance for Fitness to Practise Panels* (Council for Healthcare Regulatory Excellence, 2008*c*). This highlights the courage required to make a complaint and give evidence, especially of a sexual nature, and indicates how complainants might be supported in such cases, through the provision of advocacy and witness support. The Health Professions Council recently provided guidance to panels on cross-examination in cases of a sexual nature, so that complainants can be cross-examined only by the registrant with the complainant's written consent (Health Professions Council, 2009). The CHRE also recommends that members of fitness-to-practise panels receive appropriate training on this area as part of their induction. The CHRE is well placed to share best practice in this area, and to use its performance review framework to ensure regulators enforce the implementation of good regulatory practice.

Conclusion

The role of regulation is to protect patients. The number of fitness-to-practise cases involving boundaries, including findings of serious sexual assault, suggests that there is much more to be done to minimise professional abuse. While each element of the regulatory process has a role in minimising boundary violations, none is effective in isolation. As well as strengthening the individual components of regulation, regulators need to do more to ensure a joined-up approach across all areas of regulatory activity, to ensure, for example, that findings from fitness-to-practise cases feed into continuous improvement in education and training and inform CPD needs. While there have been some regulatory improvements, and the CHRE's Clear Sexual Boundaries project has raised the profile of this issue, there is clearly no room for complacency, as many of the recommendations made in the inquiries have yet to be implemented. Reducing prevalence requires a concerted effort by regulators, HEIs, employers and government to create a culture in which boundary violations are taken seriously. Ultimately, the capacity to minimise abuse depends on how far regulators are prepared to prioritise this vital area of patient safety, and fund it accordingly. The CHRE, as the body specifically created to ensure best practice in regulation, has a distinct role in identifying and sharing best regulatory practice, but requires the political and financial support of government to enforce standards more rigorously. Breaching professional boundaries is a fundamental violation of relationships of trust. Unless commitment to patient safety is mere rhetoric, there can surely be few areas more deserving of regulatory resources and endeavour.

References

Coe, J., Hetherington, A. & Keating, F. (2005) *A Comparison of UK Health Regulators' Guidance on Professional Boundaries.* Project Report. CHRE.

Council for Healthcare Regulatory Excellence (2008a) *Learning About Sexual Boundaries Between Healthcare Professionals and Patients: A Report on Education and Training.* CHRE. Available online at http://www.chre.org.uk/satellite/133 (accessed June 2010).

Council for Healthcare Regulatory Excellence (2008*b*) *Clear Sexual Boundaries Between Healthcare Professionals and Patients: Responsibilities of Healthcare Professionals*. CHRE. Available online at http://www.chre.org.uk/satellite/133 (accessed June 2010).

Council for Healthcare Regulatory Excellence (2008*c*) *Clear Sexual Boundaries Between Healthcare Professionals and Patients: Guidance for Fitness to Practise Panels*. CHRE. Available online at http://www.chre.org.uk/_img/pics/library/0809_harmonising_sanctions_ chre_view_FINAL_3.pdf (accessed June 2010).

Council for Healthcare Regulatory Excellence (2008*d*) *Harmonising Sanctions*. CHRE. Available online at http://www.chre.org.uk/_img/pics/library/0809_harmonising_ sanctions_chre_view_FINAL_3.pdf (accessed June 2010).

Council for Healthcare Regulatory Excellence (2009) *Guidance for Patients on Clear Sexual Boundaries with Healthcare Professionals*. CHRE. Available online at http://www.chre.org. uk/satellite/133/ (accessed June 2010).

Department of Health (2007*a*) *Safeguarding Patients*. Cm 7015. TSO (The Stationery Office). Available online at http://www.dh.gov.uk/en/Publicationsandstatistics/Publications/ PublicationsPolicyAndGuidance/DH_065953 (accessed June 2010).

Department of Health (2007*b*) *Trust, Assurance and Safety: The Regulation of Health Professionals*. Cm 7013. TSO (The Stationery Office). Available online at http://www.dh.gov.uk/en/ Publicationsandstatistics/Publications/PublicationsPolicyAndGuidance/DH_065946 (accessed June 2010).

General Medical Council (2006) *Maintaining Boundaries*. GMC. Available online at http:// www.gmc-uk.org/guidance/current/library/maintaining_boundaries.asp (accessed June 2010).

Halter, M., Brown, H. & Stone, J. (2007) *Sexual Boundary Violations by Health Employees: An Overview of the Published Empirical Literature*. Council for Healthcare Regulatory Excellence.

Health Professions Council (2009) *Practice Note: Cross-examination in Cases of a Sexual Nature*. Available online at http://www.hpc-uk.org/assets/documents/10002474PRACTICE_ NOTE_CrossExaminationinCasesofaSexualNature.pdf (accessed June 2010).

NHS Employers (2008) Clear sexual boundaries between professionals and patients. Available online at http://www.nhsemployers.org/EmploymentPolicyAndPractice/ UKEmploymentPractice/Regulation/Pages/Sexual-Boundaries.aspx (accessed June 2010).

Nursing and Midwifery Council (2009) Clear sexual boundaries. http://www.nmc-uk.org/ Nurses-and-midwives/Advice-by-topic/A/Advice/Clear-sexual-boundaries/. Accessed 20 July 2010.

Royal College of Psychiatrists (2007) *Sexual Boundary Issues in Psychiatric Settings*. College Report CR145. Royal College of Psychiatrists.

Royal Pharmaceutical Society of Great Britain (2008) *Guidance on Maintaining Clear Sexual Boundaries: Expanding on the Principles of the Code of Ethics*. RPSGB. Available online at http://www.rpsgb.org/pdfs/sexualboundariesguid.pdf (accessed June 2010).

CHAPTER 16

The role of the General Medical Council

Joan Trowell

Overview

This chapter describes the role of the General Medical Council in the regulation of the medical profession and the Council's statutory fitness-to-practise procedures current since 2004. It reviews the Kerr/Haslam Inquiry's comments and recommendations which are relevant to the role of the regulatory framework of the medical profession: the need to raise concerns about colleagues when their behaviour has placed patients at risk; and the failures of the profession to raise and consider concerns that allowed the continued abuse of patients over many years. Relevant Council guidance is highlighted and details are reviewed of cases handled in 2008 where concerns were raised about abuse of the doctor–patient relationship.

Background

The General Medical Council (GMC) is the independent regulator for doctors in the UK. Its statutory purpose is to protect, promote and maintain the health and safety of the public by ensuring proper standards in the practice of medicine. In short, it ensures that patients can have confidence in doctors. The GMC does this by:

- keeping up-to-date registers of qualified doctors
- fostering good medical practice
- promoting high standards of medical education and training
- dealing firmly and fairly with doctors whose fitness to practise is in doubt.

Such a system should:

- put patient safety at its heart
- be independent of government and of dominance by any single group
- provide an integrated regulatory framework which keeps together the GMC's four interlocking functions detailed above.

Box 16.1 Kerr/Haslam Inquiry recommendations bearing on the GMC

Among the recommendations of the report of the Kerr/Haslam Inquiry were that managers, and mental health and social care professionals must be left in no doubt that the breach of professional boundaries with regard to their patients (service users) is unacceptable, and must always be treated as harmful. Every effort must be made to prevent all patient abuse. Ways to achieve this change of ethos include:

- *Education* – of all staff at all levels – on the identification and preservation of proper boundaries, and the harm caused by boundary transgressions, commencing at undergraduate level through all the relevant professions. The message must be reinforced in induction training, in continuous professional development and through employment contracts that detail specifically unacceptable behaviour. The message must be supported by clear and enforceable codes of conduct by National Health Service trusts and by the regulatory bodies. There must be clear boundaries, clear sanctions and no tolerance of the abuse of patients.
- *Promoting the obligation to speak out*. Patient safety requires a culture where speaking out (whether or not categorised as whistle-blowing) is welcomed, where minor transgressions can be addressed at early stages and (if possible) resolved. The National Health Service must fully support its staff, who in turn must be left in no doubt that the culture of turning a blind eye is unacceptable, and that to stay silent may be to perpetuate and thus participate in wrongdoing.

Source: Department of Health (2005).

The interests of patients are best served by professionals who have ownership of the principles of good practice. However, mere assertions of professionalism have been shown to be insufficient, and public confidence in professional regulation requires active lay involvement in all the roles required and a clear framework linking the levels of professional regulation. Doctors must demonstrate to the public that they are fit to practise; with the advent of revalidation, this will become overt.

Several public inquiries into a succession of high-profile failures of doctors and of regulation led to critical scrutiny of medical regulation and the wider healthcare system (see Chapter 15). Those inquiry reports served to express the public's expectations of their relationship with their doctors, and made many recommendations (Box 16.1).

Framework of regulation

The Kerr/Haslam report (Department of Health, 2005) highlighted the link between professional regulation and workplace regulation, two of the

191

four-layer model of medical regulation that the GMC believes provides a helpful framework:

- *Personal regulation* reflects the way in which individual doctors regulate themselves, based upon their commitment to a common set of ethics.
- *Team-based regulation* reflects the increasing importance of team working and requires health professionals to take responsibility for the performance of the team.
- *Workplace regulation* reflects the responsibility that the National Health Service (NHS) and other healthcare providers have for ensuring that their employees are fit for their roles. Workplace regulation is expressed through clinical governance and performance management systems.
- *Professional regulation* in the UK is undertaken by the GMC and other statutory health regulators.

To these four national levels should be added the international level, as regulators must be able to regulate a mobile workforce and this requires better sharing of information across national boundaries. This is especially necessary in the European Union (EU), where the political priority attached to freedom of movement has attenuated, or even removed, the regulator's ability to control who is entitled to be registered. In the wider international context, the GMC has been active in this drive to coordinate regulation across international borders, and has worked with organisations such as the International Association of Medical Regulatory Authorities (IAMRA), of which it was a founding member, and the Conférence Européenne des Ordres des Médicins (CEOM).

Where local systems are effective, there is no need for the national regulator, the GMC, to duplicate local activity. Instead, the GMC as national regulator should target resources where local systems do not exist or are not effective. As the Hampton report (Hampton, 2005) explains:

If regulators operate effectively, and use the best evidence to programme their work, administrative burdens ... can be reduced while maintaining or even improving regulatory outcomes. ... Risk assessment is an essential means of directing regulatory resources where they can have the maximum impact on outcomes.

In the context of healthcare, a risk-based approach is contingent upon the existence of effective local clinical governance, and is therefore dependent on strengthening clinical governance within the NHS.

The relevance of revalidation and the licence to practise

The GMC works in partnership with others to enhance workplace regulation, to strengthen the connections between workplace and national regulation, to introduce licensing and re-licensing, and to develop re-certification as the second element of revalidation. However, if there is concern that evidence may indicate that a doctor has breached professional boundaries, colleagues should not wait for the mechanisms of clinical governance and revalidation to detect and deal with the breach. They themselves should take action. Such a concern should generally be taken forward as it arises, as a conduct issue. Nonetheless, both local clinical governance and revalidation systems will be relevant, as it could be that a complaint which was dropped as unsubstantiated, or concerns from colleagues that failed to produce any specific evidence, could be raised and brought together in appraisal, highlighting a need for further investigation or action. When events occur which by their nature involve only one doctor and one patient present at the time, patterns of behaviour become increasingly important in substantiating the evidence produced.

The GMC fitness-to-practise procedures

Until revalidation with re-licensing is implemented the GMC relies on reports to it by those at a local level, whether patients, their relatives or professional colleagues and those acting in a public capacity, such as the NHS management of the trust which employs the doctor. The GMC also receives information from the courts, the police, and local and national newspapers if a doctor is subject to criminal proceedings.

If a doctor is reported to the GMC, the procedures aim to judge the issues raised against the relevant professional guidance published by the GMC. The main priority of these procedures is to protect patients, but the procedures, which are statutory, aim to be fair to the doctors.

Since November 2004 the GMC has been able to consider issues of criminality, conduct, performance and health together, and also to take action when a doctor has been the subject of a determination by another regulatory body. The GMC additionally has the power to impose interim sanctions if this is considered necessary to protect patients. It may also act when a doctor's actions are such that they undermine public trust in the profession. These interim sanctions are imposed by the interim orders panels (IOPs) and can continue for up to 18 months while other investigations or criminal proceedings take place. The IOPs meet in private, unless the doctor asks for a public hearing, but any sanctions are included on the website in the list of registered medical practitioners.

The fitness-to-practise procedures are divided into two stages: investigation and adjudication, which involve separate staff and decision makers. An initial triage system allows any issues that can be more appropriately investigated and dealt with at a local level to be referred to the doctor's employer. If this local investigation raises serious concerns for patient safety, the matter is returned to the GMC, but otherwise the GMC plays no further part in the investigation. The triage also allows the more serious complaints to be fast-tracked and dealt with promptly.

When the GMC investigates a complaint, the holistic approach allowed since November 2004 permits appropriate assessments of the doctor's professional performance and health to be made, which can add to evidence from patients, employers and from professional colleagues. Case examiners are the key decision makers during the investigation stage. All decisions at the end of an investigation must be agreed by both a medical and a lay case examiner. Where an accusation against a doctor is referred forward for adjudication, it is heard by a fitness-to-practise panel. These panels are made up of both lay and medical panellists, who are appointed following a rigorous assessment and training process. GMC Council members are not involved in individual fitness-to-practise decisions. Eight cases investigated by GMC fitness-to-practise panels are detailed in Appendix 4, by way of illustration.

The GMC is committed to transparency in its procedures and this is reflected in the decision to hold all fitness-to-practise panel hearings in public, but there are arrangements for evidence concerning a doctor's health and any evidence from a vulnerable witness to be heard in private.

If the facts are found proved, the panel will decide whether the doctor's fitness to practise is impaired. If so, the panel has the possibility of placing sanctions on the doctor's registration; these may include conditions, suspension for up to 3 years in the first instance, or erasure of the doctor's name from the Medical Register, which is for a minimum of 5 years and normally is presumed to be for life. In certain circumstances where it is considered that the findings, if proved, could not lead to suspension, there are statutory provisions for consensual agreement to undertakings. With the doctor's agreement these undertakings may be imposed without a hearing before a fitness-to-practise panel. Undertakings have the same force and effect as conditions. Any conditions and undertakings that affect a doctor's practice are made public on the GMC website.

If at any stage the doctor's fitness to practise is found not to be impaired but there has been a significant departure from GMC guidance, the GMC may issue a warning. This does not restrict the doctor's registration but for 5 years it must be declared at appraisal and when applying for a licence to practise.

All decisions relating to a doctor's fitness to practise can be subjected to judicial review and appealed to the High Court.

GMC guidance

The GMC published core high-level guidance for doctors in *Good Medical Practice* (General Medical Council, 2006*a*), including a number of principles relevant to breaching boundaries (see Box 16.2). Further, more detailed advice on maintaining professional boundaries and raising concerns about colleagues was provided in *Maintaining Boundaries* (General Medical Council, 2006*b*) (see Box 16.3). Sexual and improper emotional relationships with current and former patients are also discussed.

Box 16.2 GMC guidelines on the duties of a doctor relevant to breaching boundaries

The following are direct quotations from different sections of *Good Medical Practice* (General Medical Council, 2006a).

- Make the care of your patient your first concern.
- Treat patients as individuals and respect their dignity.
- Treat patients politely and considerately.
- Act without delay if you have good reason to believe that you or a colleague may be putting patients at risk.
- Never abuse your patients' trust in you or the public's trust in the profession.

Maintaining trust in the profession
You must not use your professional position to establish or pursue a sexual or improper emotional relationship with a patient or someone close to them.

Conduct and performance of colleagues
You must protect patients from risk of harm posed by another colleague's conduct, performance or health. The safety of patients must come first at all times. If you have concerns that a colleague may not be fit to practise, you must take appropriate steps without delay, so that the concerns are investigated and patients protected where necessary. This means you must give an honest explanation of your concerns to an appropriate person from your employing or contracting body, and follow their procedures.

If there are no appropriate local systems, or local systems do not resolve the problem, and you are still concerned about the safety of patients, you should inform the relevant regulatory body. If you are not sure what to do, discuss your concerns with an impartial colleague or contact your defence body, a professional organisation, or the GMC for advice.

If you have management responsibilities you should make sure that systems are in place through which colleagues can raise concerns about risks to patients, and you must follow the guidance in *Management for Doctors*.

Being honest and trustworthy
You must make sure that your conduct at all times justifies your patients' trust in you and the public's trust in the profession.

There is also guidance on the particularly important professional boundary that relates to intimate examinations and the necessity for an impartial observer ('chaperone') to be present during an intimate examination (Box 16.4). Whenever a doctor examines a patient he or she should be sensitive to what the patient may perceive as intimate. This is likely to include examinations of breasts, genitalia and rectum, but could also include any examination where it is necessary to touch or even be close to the patient. By highlighting some of the issues associated with intimate examinations, the GMC does not intend to deter the doctor from carrying them out when necessary. Following this guidance and making detailed and accurate records at the time of examination, or shortly afterwards, will help to justify decisions and actions.

Box 16.3 GMC guidelines on maintaining professional boundaries

The following are direct quotations from different sections of *Maintaining Boundaries* (General Medical Council, 2006*b*).

Trust is a critical component in the doctor–patient partnership: patients must be able to trust doctors with their lives and health. In most successful doctor–patient relationships a professional boundary exists between doctor and patient. If this boundary is breached, this can undermine the patient's trust in their doctor, as well as the public's trust in the medical profession.

The doctor–patient relationship may involve an imbalance of power between the doctor and the patient. This could arise, for example, from the doctor having access to expertise and healthcare resources which the patient needs, or the possible vulnerability – emotional or physical – of a patient seeking healthcare. This may be particularly acute in some specialties such as psychiatry but can arise in any relationship between doctor and patient.

Sexual and improper emotional relationships with current and former patients:

In order to maintain professional boundaries, and the trust of patients and the public, you must not establish or pursue a sexual or improper emotional relationship with a patient. You must not use your professional relationship with a patient to establish or pursue a relationship with someone close to them. For example, you must not use home visits to pursue a relationship with a member of a patient's family.

You must not pursue a sexual relationship with a former patient, where at the time of the professional relationship the patient was vulnerable, for example because of mental health problems, or because of their lack of maturity.

Pursuing a sexual relationship with a former patient may be inappropriate, regardless of the length of time elapsed since the therapeutic relationship ended. This is because it may be difficult to be certain that the professional relationship is not being abused.

If circumstances arise in which social contact with a former patient leads to the possibility of a sexual relationship beginning, you must use your professional judgement and give careful consideration to the nature and circumstances of the relationship, taking account of the following:

- when the professional relationship ended and how long it lasted
- the nature of the previous professional relationship
- whether the patient was particularly vulnerable at the time of the professional relationship
- whether they are still vulnerable
- and whether you will be caring for other members of the patient's family.

If you are not sure whether you are – or could be seen to be – abusing your professional position, it may help to discuss your situation with an impartial colleague, a defence body, medical association or (confidentially) with a member of the GMC Standards and Ethics team.

Box 16.4 GMC guidance on intimate examinations

The following are direct quotations from different sections of *Maintaining Boundaries* (General Medical Council, 2006*b*).

Before conducting an intimate examination you should:

1 explain to the patient why an examination is necessary and give the patient an opportunity to ask questions
2 explain what the examination will involve, in a way the patient can understand, so that the patient has a clear idea of what to expect, including any potential pain or discomfort
3 obtain the patient's permission before the examination and record that permission has been obtained
4 give the patient privacy to undress and dress and keep the patient covered as much as possible to maintain their dignity. Do not assist the patient in removing clothing unless you have clarified with them that your assistance is required.

During the examination you should:

1 explain what you are going to do before you do it and, if this differs from what you have already outlined to the patient, explain why and seek the patient's permission
2 be prepared to discontinue the examination if the patient asks you to
3 keep discussion relevant and do not make unnecessary personal comments.

You must follow the guidance in *Consent: Patients and Doctors Making Decisions Together*.

Chaperones
Wherever possible, you should offer the patient the security of having an impartial observer (a 'chaperone') present during an intimate examination. This applies whether or not you are the same gender as the patient.
   A chaperone does not have to be medically qualified but will ideally:

• be sensitive, and respectful of the patient's dignity and confidentiality
• be prepared to reassure the patient if they show signs of distress or discomfort
• be familiar with the procedures involved in a routine intimate examination
• be prepared to raise concerns about a doctor if misconduct occurs.

   In some circumstances, a member of practice staff, or a relative or friend of the patient may be an acceptable chaperone.
   If either you or the patient does not wish the examination to proceed without a chaperone present, or if either of you is uncomfortable with the choice of chaperone, you may offer to delay the examination to a later date when a chaperone (or an alternative chaperone) will be available, if this is compatible with the patient's best interests.
   You should record any discussion about chaperones and its outcome. If a chaperone is present, you should record that fact and make a note of their identity. If the patient does not want a chaperone, you should record that the offer was made and declined.

Box 16.5 GMC guidance about sexualised behaviour and duty to report

The following is directly quoted from *Maintaining Boundaries* (General Medical Council, 2006*b*).

In order to maintain professional boundaries and the trust of patients and the public you must never make a sexual advance towards a patient nor display 'sexualised behaviour'. Sexualised behaviour has been defined as 'acts, words or behaviour designed or intended to arouse or gratify sexual impulses and desires'.

If you have grounds to believe that a colleague has, or may have, demonstrated sexualised behaviour when with a patient, you must take appropriate steps without delay so that your concerns are investigated and patients protected where necessary. Where there is a suspicion that a sexual assault or other criminal activity has taken place, it should be reported to the police.

Guidance on steps you should take is included in *Good Medical Practice*, in *Management for Doctors* and in the supplementary guidance, *Raising Concerns About Patient Safety*.

If you are not sure what to do, discuss your concerns with an impartial colleague or contact your defence body, a professional organisation or the GMC for advice.

You should respect patient confidentiality wherever possible when reporting your concerns. Nevertheless, the safety of patients must come first at all times and therefore takes precedence over maintaining confidentiality. If you are satisfied that it is necessary to identify the patient, wherever practical you should seek the patient's consent to disclosure of any information and, if this is refused, inform the patient of your intention to disclose the information.

In all cases where a patient reports a breach of sexual boundaries, appropriate support and assistance must be offered to the patient. All such reports must be properly investigated, whatever the apparent credibility of the patient.

If a patient displays sexualised behaviour, wherever possible treat them politely and considerately and try to re-establish a professional boundary. If you should find it necessary to end the professional relationship you must follow the guidance *Good Medical Practice*.

Specific consent, usually in writing, is required for the intimate examination of anaesthetised patients and for any intimate examination performed by a student.

The GMC has published specific guidance about 'sexualised behaviour' (which has been defined as 'acts, words or behaviour designed or intended to arouse or gratify sexual impulses and desires') and also a doctor's duty to report such behaviour (see Box 16.5).

GMC guidance relating to medical students

In view of the emphasis placed by the report of the Kerr/Haslam Inquiry on education and training, it is relevant to mention the GMC guidance on professional boundaries that relates to medical students.

Box 16.6 GMC guidance relating to students on professional boundaries

The following two paragraphs are quoted from different sections of *Medical Students: Professional Behaviour and Fitness to Practise* (General Medical Council, 2009).

Medical students will have extensive contact with patients during their medical course. Although there are limits to these clinical encounters and students are supervised, patients may consider the student to be in a position of responsibility, and so may attach added importance to their opinions or comments.

Doctors and students are expected to maintain a professional boundary between themselves and their patients or anyone close to the patient. They must not use their professional position to cause distress or to exploit patients.

Although the GMC does not register or regulate medical students, it does control entry to the register and oversees the content and standard of medical education in university medical schools in Great Britain. In this capacity the GMC has issued guidance which emphasises that whenever they are relating to patients, medical students must be supervised, and has issued guidance for those responsible for supervising students (see Box 16.6).

Procedural changes over time

The GMC has evolved ever since it was founded by the Medical Act of 1858, as have the GMC's fitness-to-practise procedures, which are governed by statute. This evolution accelerated after the 'Health Procedures' were introduced in the 1970s and the 'Performance Procedures' in the 1990s. Over the 10 years that followed the implementation of these changes it became apparent that this piecemeal reform had created procedural complications that led to practical problems for the GMC when considering concerns raised about doctors. At the same time, and paralleling the rise in the voice of the consumer, lay members of Council were appointed in increasing numbers from the 1970s, and patients became more vocal in complaining about their doctors. Finally, from the late 1990s several major scandals emerged involving the NHS and the medical profession and led to formal public inquiries.

The changes introduced to professional regulation in response to the reports of these inquiries and to the changing views of society included a reduction in the size of the Council; reform of the fitness-to-practise procedures – in particular allowing the doctor's conduct, professional performance and health all to be investigated concurrently; the separation of the investigatory stage; and the use of separate trained decision makers, who were not Council members, both during the investigation and on the fitness-to-practise panels. As a result of these changes, the procedures also ceased to consider serious professional misconduct, but considered instead if the doctor's fitness to practise was impaired to such an extent that in order to protect the public it was necessary to place restrictions on the doctor's professional registration. These reformed procedures were introduced from November 2004, on the basis of parliamentary legislation passed in 2003, preceding the Kerr/Haslam Inquiry, which took evidence in private and continued meeting up to December 2004 and did not report till 2005.

A further development in the regulatory scene has been the statutory introduction in 2003 of the Council for the Regulation of Healthcare Professionals (CRHP), which changed its name to the Council for Healthcare Regulatory Excellence (CHRE) in 2005. This has an important coordinating role in identifying and promoting best practice among the healthcare regulatory bodies, and has sought to impose some uniformity in the procedures and standards of the nine healthcare regulatory bodies (see Chapter 15, p. 187). It also has the power to appeal decisions which it considers to be too lenient, while doctors can also appeal if they consider the outcome to be too harsh. Initially, the CHRE did make several such appeals on the outcomes of fitness-to-practise panels, some from the GMC, that related to professional boundaries, normally when the initial sanction had been suspension of the doctor's registration and the court (High Court of Justice, Queen's Bench Division Administrative Court) was asked to consider whether the verdict should have been erasure. Outcomes of these appeals were mixed, but the actions of the CHRE reinforced the importance of observing professional boundaries. At the time of writing, no appeals had been initiated by the CHRE since 2006.

Changes to guidance over time

The GMC considers it necessary to observe boundaries in professional relationships. This was reflected in the early guidance, the 'Blue Book', which attempted to outline those activities which were deemed to be unbefitting in a medical practitioner. This was replaced in 1993 with the first edition of *Good Medical Practice*, which, for the first time, set out in simple and accessible language the principles of good practice expected of every doctor.

Good Medical Practice has been revised since 1993 and included guidance on the conduct of intimate examinations from 2000. The trend has been for increasingly detailed guidance and since the report of the Kerr/Haslam Inquiry this has included *Maintaining Boundaries* (General Medical Council, 2006b).

The CHRE has also published guidance on sexual boundaries between healthcare professionals and patients (Council for Healthcare Regulatory Excellence, 2008). As this applies to the nine professional regulators dealing with healthcare professionals, it contains some details not relevant to doctors but, where relevant, does not differ from the guidance published by the GMC and current GMC practice.

Data collection

The statutory obligations are for the GMC to hold a register of properly qualified medical practitioners, to include their registered medical qualification, and an address at which they can be contacted. More recently, the GMC has also collected information on the gender of the doctor and has recently added information on the doctor's date of birth, ethnicity and specialty of medical practice. The data collection with the previous fitness-to-practise procedures included only whether the issues arose from convictions, conduct, professional performance or health concerns. With the introduction of the reformed procedures more detail is recorded, as several different issues can be investigated concurrently; as information technology (IT) has evolved, so has the GMC's ability to analyse the details of the concerns about doctors that are reported to it. The most recent changes in the GMC IT system have been rolled out since 2006, and these made possible the more detailed analysis from 2008, although comparison with the past is not possible.

The total number of referrals made to the GMC in 2008 was 5195. There were 52 complaints (about 47 individual doctors) where one or many allegations (68 in all) related to an improper relationship with a patient. Of these, 22 doctors were referred for a hearing, of which 5 doctors were still awaiting hearing in November 2009, pending the outcome of criminal proceedings. Of those cases heard, 5 doctors were found not to have impaired fitness to practise, while 12 were found to be impaired. Of these, 8 were erased and 4 suspended. (See also Chapter 13 on regulatory sanctions, p. 155.)

Conclusion

The doctor–patient relationship is central to the trust that must underpin all medical practice. Doctors have a relationship with patients that is among the most intimate that individuals allow and society accepts, and is certainly more intimate than allowed outside those with a close sexual or family relationship. It is an unequal relationship, and as such the onus is on the doctor to maintain appropriate boundaries. To abuse these boundaries undermines the trust that patients place in the medical profession.

The GMC considers that any concerns about such abuse should be investigated, but the fitness-to-practise procedures rely on people who know of such abuses to report their concerns. Acting as a whistle-blower requires courage and a clear understanding of appropriate professional behaviour, and whistle-blowers, whether doctors or patients, should be supported by the medical and other healthcare professions and the NHS, as to fail to do this can have serious consequences not only for the patient involved but more widely, throughout the medical profession.

References

Council for Healthcare Regulatory Excellence (2008) *Clear Sexual Boundaries Between Healthcare Professionals and Patients: Responsibilities of Healthcare Professionals.* CHRE.

Department of Health (2005) *The Kerr/Haslam Inquiry.* TSO (The Stationery Office).

General Medical Council (2006a) *Good Medical Practice.* London: GMC.

General Medical Council (2006b) *Maintaining Boundaries.* GMC.

General Medical Council (2009) *Medical Students: Professional Behaviour and Fitness to Practise.* GMC.

Hampton, P. (2005) *Reducing Administrative Burdens: Effective Inspection and Enforcement* (the Hampton report). HM Treasury.

Extract from *Vulnerable Patients, Safe Doctors*

The following is taken from *Vulnerable Patients, Safe Doctors: Good Practice in Our Clinical Relationships* (Royal College of Psychiatrists, College Report CR146, 2007). Although the boundaries of the psychiatric encounter are described below, the principles hold for boundaries of all doctor–patient encounters and similarly for the avoidance of boundary violations.

Boundaries of the psychiatric encounter

A number of features help to provide the boundaries of the psychiatric professional encounter, all of which are the responsibility of the psychiatrist. These include:

- setting (hospital, clinic, care home or family home)
- time (usually within agreed service hours)
- duration (agreed and consistently maintained)
- use of appropriate professional language
- appropriate professional dress and insignia
- limited and socially sanctioned physical touch
- the patient's mental health needs, not social or sexual needs, being taken as paramount.

There is clear evidence that even minor violations of these boundaries may be damaging to patients. Some are unacceptable in any circumstances, while others are not always clearly harmful to patients. Even those not unequivocally harmful should raise questions for the doctor or patient about their appropriateness, but may not be finally judged except in their detailed context.

The commonest boundary violations are non-sexual, and include inappropriate self-disclosure, involving the patient in a dual role (e.g. employing a patient or a patient's relative), speaking aggressively or rudely to patients and financial exploitation. Sexual violations are less common, but often start with apparently minor boundary violations, such as unjustifiably prolonged sessions, appointments out of working hours, treatment outside the normal place of work, except where clinically justified, and (in private practice) not charging a fee. Sexual boundary violations between psychiatrists and their patients usually take place in the context of a 'special relationship', to which the patient 'assents' rather than consents; they usually come to light when the relationship ends and the patient then reports the unprofessional relationship. The General Medical Council sees sexual boundary violations by doctors as serious professional misconduct and will normally remove the doctor from the medical register.

Avoiding boundary violations: a practice guide

- Sexual relationships with patients or former patients are unethical and unacceptable.
- Physical touch beyond normal social exchange should be used with caution. A 'no touch' policy is unworkable and may be anti-therapeutic, but the inherent power imbalance between professionals and patients means that touch of any kind may be misinterpreted.
- Inappropriate self-disclosure (the commonest form of boundary violation) or disclosure of confidential personal material without consent should be avoided. Psychiatrists should make themselves familiar with the guidance on confidentiality produced by the Royal College of Psychiatrists (2006).
- Treatment or therapy should generally not take place in a practitioner's home. If the practitioner is in private practice and works from home, the work should take place in a designated area, kept apart from the practitioner's ordinary domiciliary arrangements.
- Treatment or therapy should not generally take place outside the workplace (e.g. in restaurants or places of entertainment).
- Treatment, therapy or clinical assessment in the patient's home is justified only on clinical grounds, and clinicians should be prepared to justify how and why such work has taken place.
- Treatment or therapy outside in-patient settings should generally take place within working hours of the service (which may vary). If such work is to take place at unusual hours, this should be agreed with a mentor, supervisor or senior colleague and the reasons recorded.
- All psychiatrists should have a named supervisor, clinical manager or senior colleague with whom they can discuss their work.
- For more intensive work, such as formal psychodynamic psychotherapy, or work with patients with complex needs (especially Axis II disorders), supervision is essential and practitioners will have to justify why they did not have an identified supervisor if they fail to do so and their work is questioned.
- Psychiatrists should avoid being in dual roles with patients, for example being both the responsible medical officer (RMO) and psychotherapist.

As stated in *Good Medical Practice* (General Medical Council, 2006), psychiatrists should avoid treating family members, friends, family of friends, colleagues or family of colleagues. This is particularly true in cases where the patient is a doctor (e.g. a fellow psychiatrist).

- Other role conflicts include issues relating to money and dual relationships. Psychiatrists should not appear as expert or professional witnesses in cases where they know the patient in a psychotherapeutic relationship. They may act as professional witnesses but will be bound by their duty of confidentiality in the ordinary way (see Royal College of Psychiatrists, 2006). There are rare occasions (usually in forensic psychiatry) where the RMO can also act as an expert witness as well as a professional witness. In such cases, the RMO needs to consider the legal questions carefully and advise the court of a possible conflict of interest. Junior staff should not be placed in situations of role conflict.

References

General Medical Council (2006) *Good Medical Practice* (4th edn). General Medical Council, http://www.gmc-uk.org/guidance/good_medical_practice/index.asp.

Royal College of Psychiatrists (2006) *Good Psychiatric Practice: Confidentiality and Information Sharing* (Council Report CR133). Royal College of Psychiatrists, http://www.rcpsych.ac.uk/publications/collegereports/cr/cr133.aspx.

Codes of ethics of psychiatric associations in other countries

Canadian Psychiatric Association: position statement on sexual misconduct

The four points quoted below comprise the position statement submitted by the Professional Standards and Practice Council to the Board of Directors of the Canadian Psychiatric Association and was approved in 1995, when it replaced 1985 statement (online at http://publications.cpa-apc.org/media.php?mid=188&xwm=true).

- The Canadian Psychiatric Association deems sexual activity of any kind between a psychiatrist and his or her patient to be sexual misconduct and unacceptable in any circumstances.
- The Canadian Psychiatric Association deems any form of sexualisation by the psychiatrist of the psychiatrist–patient relationship to be unethical.
- The Canadian Psychiatric Association presumes sexual relationships with former patients to be unethical.
- Any member of the Canadian Psychiatric Association losing a medical licence as a result of sexual misconduct will have his or her membership in the Association revoked.

American Psychiatric Association: 'Principles of medical ethics'

The four points quoted below are taken from 'Principles of medical ethics, with annotations especially applicable to psychiatry', published by the American Psychiatric Association in November 2003 as an amended edition of a document first published in 2001:

- The requirement that the physician conduct himself/herself with propriety in his or her profession and in all the actions of his or her life is especially important in the case of the psychiatrist because the patient tends to model his or her behavior after that of his or her psychiatrist by identification.

- Further, the necessary intensity of the treatment relationship may tend to activate sexual and other needs and fantasies on the part of both patient and psychiatrist, while weakening the objectivity necessary for control.
- Additionally, the inherent inequality in the doctor–patient relationship may lead to exploitation of the patient.
- Sexual activity with a current or former patient is unethical.

Royal Australian and New Zealand College of Psychiatrists: Ethical Guideline number 8

The points quoted below are from 'Sexual relationships with patients', published as Ethical Guideline number 8 by the Royal Australian and New Zealand College of Psychiatrists in August 2005 (GC2005/3 R25):

- Psychiatrists, like other medical practitioners, are required to adhere strictly to their ethical obligations. In psychiatry there is an even stronger obligation to avoid exploitation because of the more intensive therapeutic relationship with patients, and the powerful emotional forces often released during treatment.
- Psychiatrists face certain inescapable duties. They must be competent technically and watchful to ensure that whatever happens in therapy is in the patient's best interests. Psychiatrists should be aware of the need to monitor not only the patient's emotions but their own, in the interests of the therapeutic process and for the patient's benefit. This firmly excludes any exploitation of the patient sexually, financially or in any other way.
- Sexual relationships between current and former patients and their psychiatrists are never acceptable and constitute unethical behaviour. The term 'sexual relationship' is not restricted to sexual intercourse. In this guideline, sexual relationship includes: any behaviour, including discussion, which has as its purpose some form of sexual gratification, or which might reasonably be construed as having that purpose.

Guidance from the Council for Healthcare Regulatory Excellence

Extract from *Clear Sexual Boundaries Between Healthcare Professionals and Patients: Responsibilities of Healthcare Professionals* (CHRE, 2008; http://www.chre.org.uk/_img/pics/library/0801_Clear_Sexual_boundaries_professionals.pdf).

Examples of sexualised behaviour by healthcare professionals towards patients or their carers:
- asking for or accepting a date
- sexual humour during consultations or examinations
- inappropriate sexual or demeaning comments, or asking clinically irrelevant questions, for example about their body or underwear, sexual performance or sexual orientation
- requesting details of sexual orientation, history or preferences that are not necessary or relevant
- internal examination without gloves
- asking for, or accepting an offer of, sex
- watching a patient undress (unless a justified part of an examination)
- unnecessary exposure of the patient's body
- accessing a patient's or family member's records to find out personal information not clinically required for their treatment
- unplanned home visits with sexual intent
- taking or keeping photographs of the patient or their family that are not clinically necessary
- telling patients about their own sexual problems, preferences or fantasies, or disclosing other intimate personal details
- clinically unjustified physical examinations
- intimate examinations carried out without the patient's explicit consent
- continuing with examination or treatment when consent has been refused or withdrawn
- any sexual act induced by the healthcare professional for their own sexual gratification
- the exchange of drugs or services for sexual favours
- exposure of parts of the healthcare professional's body to the patient
- sexual assault.

Examples of determinations by the General Medical Council's Fitness to Practise Panels

The following eight cases, supplied by the GMC, were heard by Fitness to Practise Panels and the final determinations are given in full. They are included here to give real-life examples of doctors who breached boundaries and the GMC principles of *Good Medical Practice* (GMP). The GMC advises that it does not give clear thresholds between acceptable and unacceptable behaviour: each case which comes before a Fitness to Practise Panel is judged on its own merits and assessed on the particular circumstances of the case.

Cases 1 and 2 led to 12 months' suspension from the Medical Register; cases 3–8 led to erasure.

Case 1

Summary

The doctor was admonished by a Medical Council outside the UK for pursuing an inappropriate relationship with a vulnerable psychiatric patient.

Relevant paragraphs of Good Medical Practice

The case relates to the *Relationships with patients* section of GMP, specifically paragraph 32 on maintaining trust in the profession. It also relates to the *Probity* section, specifically paragraphs 56 and 57 on being honest and trustworthy.

Determination on impaired fitness to practise

The Panel has now considered, on the basis of facts found proved, whether Dr X's fitness to practise is impaired, pursuant to section 35C(2)(e) of the Medical Act 1983 as amended, namely by reason of a determination by the

X Medical Council to the effect that his actions amounted to professional misconduct.

The Panel has given detailed consideration to the evidence submitted, based upon the transcripts of the proceedings before the X Medical Council on [date]. It has noted the contents of text messages which passed between Dr X in [date] and a patient, Ms T, who had been under his care for a considerable period of time up to the termination of his contract in [date]. It also took account of the correspondence between Dr X and the X Medical Council and the report by Dr L [date] which was submitted to the X Medical Council Fitness to Practise Committee. The Panel has heard and accepts the evidence of Ms T's extreme vulnerability as a consequence of her social, medical and psychiatric history. That vulnerability would have been known to Dr X, even if he was not fully aware of the entirety of her history.

The Panel has had regard to the General Medical Council's (GMC's) documents, 'Good Medical Practice' (May 2001) and those parts of the 'Indicative Sanctions Guidance' which relate to the issue of impairment. The guidance also indicates that one of the GMC's functions exercised through its Fitness to Practise Panels is to protect patients, maintain public confidence in the profession and to declare and uphold proper standards of professional behaviour.

'Good Medical Practice' states, under the heading 'The duties of a doctor registered with the General Medical Council', that: 'patients must be able to trust doctors with their lives and well-being. ... In particular as a doctor you must respect patients' dignity...' and '... avoid abusing your position as a doctor'.

'Indicative Sanctions Guidance' makes clear that occasional one off mistakes are unlikely in themselves to indicate a fitness to practise problem. However, 'Good Medical Practice' states that 'serious or persistent failures to meet the standards in this booklet may put your registration at risk'. Furthermore, doctors occupy a position of privilege and trust in society; have access to vulnerable patients; and are expected to act with integrity and in the best interests of their patients.

The Panel has taken account of the information regarding Ms T's propensity to form inappropriately dependent relationships with those who provided care for her. It does not consider that this excuses Dr X's behaviour in pursuing an emotional and/or sexual relationship. Although Ms T was no longer under Dr X's direct care at the time, it was his responsibility to ensure that the proper doctor–patient relationship was maintained. This applied even during a period which Dr X described as one of great personal stress for him. Furthermore, the sexual nature of the text messages sent by Dr X to the patient, especially in view of her vulnerability, seriously damages the reputation of the profession as a whole and undermines public confidence.

Therefore, on the evidence adduced, the Panel finds that Dr X's fitness to practise is impaired.

Case 2

Summary

After having a consultation with a vulnerable female patient, the doctor – a psychiatrist – gave her his personal mobile phone number and called her a number of times. In another position, the doctor downloaded and stored sexual images on a computer during working hours.

Relevant paragraphs of Good Medical Practice

The case relates to the *Relationships with patients* section of GMP, specifically paragraph 32 on maintaining trust in the profession. It also relates to the *Probity* section, specifically paragraph 57 on being honest and trustworthy.

Determination on impaired fitness to practise

Dr X: at the outset of the hearing you admitted all of the factual allegations in the case. In considering whether your fitness to practise is impaired, the Panel has borne in mind these admissions, the documentary evidence submitted, Ms B's submissions on behalf of the GMC, and Mr S's submissions on your behalf.

The Panel has heard that at all material times you were a UK registered medical practitioner; and between [dates] you worked as a Senior House Officer (SHO) in Psychiatry, with the X Mental Health NHS Trust.

On [date], Patient A was admitted to X Hospital ('the Hospital') following an attempted overdose. That evening, you saw Patient A, in your capacity as duty SHO, on the Ward in the Hospital.

Patient A was discharged from the Hospital on X and was referred to the X Centre, X, for further treatment for her depression. On [date], Patient A attended an appointment with you at the X Centre. That evening you telephoned a third party, requested the third party to ask Patient A to contact you on your mobile telephone, and gave your mobile telephone number to the third party. Later the same evening, Patient A returned your call and you asked if you could call her back in a few minutes. You called Patient A back on her home telephone number. During the telephone conversation you told Patient A, that you would like to take her out for a cup of tea, that you were making an unofficial call, that you had experienced strong feelings for Patient A since your meeting with her earlier that day at the X Centre, and asked Patient A if she was disturbed by your telephone call.

On [date], you telephoned Patient A's home telephone number, from your mobile telephone, on five occasions. Patient A did not answer any of these calls and you did not speak to Patient A. On [date] you telephoned Patient A's home telephone, from your mobile telephone, on one occasion. Patient A did not answer this call and you did not speak to Patient A.

You have admitted, and the Panel has found proved that your actions were inappropriate and not in the best interests of Patient A. You admitted your personal contact with Patient A during a meeting with Dr B on [date], at a Trust disciplinary hearing held on [date].

Between [dates] you were working as a locum Staff Grade Psychiatrist with the X Mental Health NHS Trust ('the Trust') in the Adult Learning Disabilities Service. On [date], you confirmed in writing that you had read and understood the 'Computer Users – IM&T Security Responsibilities & Checklist' and the Trust's Code of Conduct.

Between [dates] via the computer provided for you by the Trust, you gained access to the internet during your hours of clinical duty. You sought websites displaying material of a sexual nature, from which you downloaded, stored, filed and categorised images of a sexual nature which were not related to your clinical practice, but were for your own gratification. You have admitted and the Panel has found proved that your actions were inappropriate, contrary to the Trust's Code of Conduct, a misuse of your Trust computer and liable to bring the profession into disrepute.

The Panel has considered, on the basis of the allegations found proved, whether your fitness to practise is impaired by reason of your misconduct. In doing so, it has taken into account the written evidence before it, which included the witness statements of a number of Trust employees involved in the two instances of alleged misconduct, copies of the images viewed and a screenshot of files from your computer. The question of impairment of fitness to practise is a matter for this Panel exercising its own judgement.

In addition, the Panel has had sight of the Trust's Code of Conduct, Information Security Policy and minutes of meetings within the Trust including your disciplinary hearing at the conclusion of which you were summarily dismissed for gross misconduct. It notes with concern your attempts, when interviewed, to explain your misconduct by reason of external circumstances, both domestic and cultural. It deplores the priority you gave to your own future career over the potential impact your misconduct could have had on Patient A's mental health.

The Panel has considered Good Medical Practice (May 2001 edition) at the time of both events. In relation to the duties of a doctor registered with the GMC, this states that: 'Patients must be able to trust doctors with their lives and well-being. To justify this trust, we as a profession have a duty to maintain a good standard of practice and care. … In particular as a doctor you must: make the care of your patient your first concern and avoid abusing your position as a doctor'. It further states, at paragraph 20: 'You must not allow your personal relationships to undermine the trust which patients place in you. In particular, you must not use your professional position to establish or pursue a sexual or improper emotional relationship with a patient'.

The Royal College of Psychiatrists publication: Good Psychiatric Practice, 2000, on page 7, states that: 'Psychiatrists need … to pay particular attention to issues concerning patients' vulnerability and to be aware of the risks of over or inappropriate involvement with their patients'. It also states that: 'Good practice will include: Paying particular attention to the doctor–patient relationship; Paying particular attention to boundaries, time and place, and being sensitive to the psychological implications of transgressing boundaries'.

The Panel has also borne in mind the Indicative Sanctions Guidance Page S3-14 and S3-15, paragraph 58, which states that: 'A question of impaired fitness to practise is likely to arise if … [a] doctor has abused a patient's trust or violated a patient's autonomy or other fundamental rights'. It further states at paragraph 11 (S1-2): 'Neither the Act nor the Rules define what is meant by impaired fitness to practice but … it is clear that the GMC's role in relation to fitness to practise is to consider concerns which are so serious as to raise the question whether the doctor concerned should continue to practise either with restrictions on registration or at all'.

In relation to Patient A, the Panel is concerned by the reckless disregard you demonstrated for her welfare in spite of your professional training and position as SHO. You knew her to be a highly vulnerable patient suffering from depression, in part at least as a result of a serious relationship breakdown. It considers that the consequences of your failure to respect boundaries towards Patient A in this regard had the potential to cause her serious harm. Instead of making the care of the patient your first concern, you pursued your own self-interest heedless of the consequences for her. This amounted to an abuse of your position, and conduct falling far below the standard expected of a registered medical practitioner.

In relation to the downloading of images the Panel has seen evidence that your behaviour related to a large number garnered systematically over a two-month period during working hours and between patient appointments. It constituted an abuse of your position as a doctor and of Trust resources and time. You viewed, downloaded, stored and filed sexually inappropriate images, demonstrating a lack of respect for the privacy and dignity of women. The Panel rejects your assertions at the Trust disciplinary hearing that your clinical practice and this activity were unrelated. Further this misuse was in contravention of 'The Computer Users IM&T Security Responsibilities & Checklist' and the Trust's Code of Conduct, which states: 'Using the Trust's facilities to access internet sites or to download material deemed by the Trust to be offensive, obscene or indecent is forbidden'.

The Panel notes that lay employees of the Trust became aware of your computer misuse and so your behaviour in this context undermined public confidence in the profession.

The public are entitled to feel able to place their trust in doctors and to have confidence that they will act honourably and with integrity. Your deliberate failures in this regard have undermined such confidence.

By your actions you have undermined the public trust and confidence in the profession and have brought the profession into disrepute. You have breached many of the fundamental principles contained within both the GMC's guidance 'Good Medical Practice' and the Royal College of Psychiatrists' guidance 'Good Psychiatric Practice'.

The Panel has a duty to act in the public interest, which includes, among other things, the protection of patients, the maintenance of public confidence in the profession and the declaring and upholding of proper standards of conduct and behaviour of the medical profession.

In view of these serious instances of misconduct, the Panel has found that your fitness to practise is impaired. The Panel has therefore determined that by reason of the facts found proved, your fitness to practise is impaired because of your misconduct.

Case 3

Summary

The doctor inappropriately touched patients whilst sedating them.

Relevant paragraphs of Good Medical Practice

This case relates to the Relationships with patients section of Good Medical Practice, specifically paragraph 21b on *The doctor–patient partnership* and paragraph 32 on *Maintaining trust in the profession*. It also relates to the Probity section, specifically paragraph 57 on *Being honest and trustworthy*.

Determination on impaired fitness to practise

Dr X, the Panel has given detailed consideration to the submissions made by Ms N on behalf of the General Medical Council and those made by Mr B on your behalf. It has noted and accepted the advice of the Legal Assessor.

The Panel has considered on the basis of the allegations found proved, whether your fitness to practise is impaired pursuant to Section 35C (2) (a) of The Medical Act 1983, as amended, by reason of your misconduct.

At all material times you were working on a consultancy basis as an anaesthetist for X Dental, whose registered office is in X. You supplied conscious sedation to dental patients at their clinics, including the X Dental Practice, X and the X Dental Centre.

In or around [date], Ms A, the manager of X Dental received a number of complaints from members of staff. These included Nurse A and Nurse B, both employed as nurses at the X Dental Practice, and from Dentist A, a dentist at the X Dental Practice. It was alleged that you had touched male patients on their stomachs, legs and genital area whilst those patients were undergoing sedation. As a result of the above complaints Ms A advised you as to your future conduct and in particular explained that the areas from the neck to the knees were 'no touch zones'.

In [date], whilst providing sedation to Patient A aged 16, at the X Dental Practice, you touched Patient A on his bare stomach, thus failing to follow the policy of 'no touch zones' as agreed with Ms A. The panel did not hear any evidence from Patient A, Patient A's mother or Nurse C that on any occasion you touched Patient A in his genital area whilst he was undergoing sedation.

On or about [date], as a result of a further complaint from a member of staff, Nurse C, a nurse employed at the X Dental Practice, you were issued with a final written warning by Ms A concerning your conduct in touching male patients and the need to practise 'no touch zones' was re-emphasised.

On [date], at the X Dental Centre, you provided conscious sedation to Patient B aged 15. Whilst Patient B was undergoing sedation you stroked his leg, rubbed his stomach, touched his genital area and cupped his genitals in your hand. Whilst Patient B was in recovery you rubbed him on his stomach. In touching Patient B you failed to follow the instructions of Ms A relating to 'no touch zones', and this was inappropriate.

Your conduct in touching and cupping Patient B's genitals was inappropriate, sexually motivated and an abuse of your professional position.

Nurse A, Nurse B, Nurse C and Dentist A all explained to the Panel that they had seen you touch the genital area of male patients inappropriately on several occasions. The Panel has also heard how you would treat female and male patients differently and that you never touched female patients other than in a professional manner. You behaved differently with certain male patients. You have stated that at times there was a need to hold the patient's contra-lateral hand in order to comfort him. This would then leave both your hand and the patient's hand lying on the patient's abdomen. You stated that any touching of the genitals would have occurred when holding the contra-lateral hand in this way and would have been inadvertent, due for example to your turning around to look at the monitor, or when the dentist lowered the patient in the dental chair. The Panel does not accept your explanation of the need to hold the contra-lateral hand. Neither does it accept that the touching of the patient's genitals was inadvertent.

The Panel is concerned to note that you continued with this type of behaviour even after you had been warned as to your future conduct.

The Panel has heard how you would rub the stomachs of male patients, over or under their clothing, and you explained that this was to comfort patients. Dr B, a Consultant Anaesthetist, called as an expert witness on behalf of the GMC in his report of [date] stated that: 'Sometimes it is helpful, mostly in children for the sedationist to put an arm around the shoulder of the patient and to give the odd squeeze … beyond that it is normally never necessary to touch either the torso or the thighs of the patient'.

In his evidence Dr B gave his opinion that patting or rubbing a patient's abdomen would be wrong.

The Panel is extremely concerned about your behaviour in general and particularly what they have found proved in regard to Patient B. The Panel found the evidence of Patient B and his mother credible and convincing. The Panel found your actions to be inappropriate, sexually motivated and an abuse of your professional position. This is a matter of serious concern.

Patient B was vulnerable as he was consciously sedated and only 15 years of age when you touched his genital area and cupped his genitals in your hand. Your behaviour not only discredits you but also undermines the confidence which the public are entitled to have in the integrity of members of the medical profession.

The Panel notes that these events took place over a period of time and your behaviour towards some male patients was complained about at two different dental clinics and at different times in [dates]. In this regard the Panel found the evidence of Nurse A, Nurse B and Dentist A credible and convincing. No evidence was adduced that either Patient B or his mother were aware of the previous complaints when they complained in [date].

The Panel has borne in mind the need to protect the public interest, which includes the maintenance of public confidence in the profession, and declaring and upholding proper standards of conduct and behaviour.

The GMC publication Good Medical Practice (May 2001) which was applicable at the time of these events states that doctors must respect their patients' privacy and dignity and must avoid abusing their position as a doctor. Your conduct was in breach of these fundamental principles.

The GMC's Indicative Sanctions Guidance at S3-15 paragraph 58 states that: 'Conduct, which shows that a doctor has acted without regard for patients' rights or feelings, or has abused their professional position as a doctor, will usually give rise to questions about a doctor's fitness to practise'.

The Panel is satisfied that your conduct has fallen below the standard that the public is entitled to expect from a registered medical practitioner.

Case 4

Summary

The doctor pursued and established a sexual relationship with a patient, administering contraceptive treatment to her despite her reluctance to undergo such treatment.

The doctor was also convicted of indecent assault on another patient, after violating boundaries during the course of a medico-legal examination.

The doctor also failed to comply with requirements made by his primary care trust in relation to chaperoning arrangements.

Relevant paragraphs of Good Medical Practice

The case relates to the *Relationships with patients* section of GMP, specifically paragraph 21b on the doctor–patient partnership, paragraph 22a on good communication and paragraph 32 on maintaining trust in the profession. It also relates to the *Probity* section, specifically paragraphs 56 and 57 on being honest and trustworthy.

Determination on impaired fitness to practise

At all material times, Dr X was a fully registered medical practitioner and worked as a General Practitioner at the X Heath Centre. Dr X was the General Practitioner for Patient A. From about [date], Dr X pursued and established a personal relationship with Patient A. The relationship with Patient A lasted until about [date]. The Panel has found that Dr X's relationship with Patient A was sexual, improper and an abuse of his professional position.

During the course of his relationship with Patient A, the Panel has found that Dr X prescribed and administered contraceptive treatment to her, knowing that she was reluctant to undergo any such treatment. In this respect the Panel found that Dr X's actions were inappropriate, and particularly as the purpose was to facilitate his sexual relationship with Patient A.

On [date], Patient B attended the X Health Centre in order to consult Dr X in relation to a medico-legal report in connection with a road traffic accident. On [date], at X Crown Court, Dr X was convicted upon indictment of one count of indecent assault on a female, namely Patient B, contrary to section 14 of the Sexual Offences Act 1956, in relation to the events of [date], during the course of Patient B's consultation with Dr X. His Honour Judge Y sentenced Dr X to nine months imprisonment.

The Panel has found that on or about [date], Dr X was informed by the X City Primary Care Trust (the Trust) that he was requested to be chaperoned when consulting and examining all females and that compliance with this would be monitored. Furthermore, it stated that documentary evidence would need to be kept in patients' records for monitoring purposes. This was conveyed to Dr X in a letter from Dr Z, the Trust GP Clinical Governance Lead, [date]. Dr X failed to comply with the requirements made by the Trust in relation to the provision of chaperones and the monitoring of that provision.

Good Medical Practice states that doctors must avoid abusing their position as a doctor. The GMC's publication 'Good Medical Practice', 1998 edition, provides guidance to doctors about relationships with patients. Good Medical Practice states as follows: 'You must do your best to establish and maintain a relationship of trust with your patients.' 'You must not use your position to establish improper personal relationships with patients, or their close relatives'.

Dr X, in pursuing a personal and sexual relationship with Patient A, crossed far beyond the boundaries of a proper doctor/patient relationship and, in this respect, abused his position.

Whilst the Panel notes that the relationship which occurred between Dr X and Patient A was consensual, it does not detract from the fact that Dr X acted wholly unprofessionally towards her. The Panel found that Patient A was a vulnerable patient and that Dr X was aware of this as he had referred her for counselling.

In relation to Patient B, Dr X crossed acceptable boundaries during the course of a medico-legal examination. Dr X was charged with, and subsequently convicted of, indecent assault on Patient B. The Panel noted the sentencing remarks of Judge Y, who stated, 'It is true that the actual indecent assaults, as it were, by themselves, are towards the lower end of the scale. There are many cases of indecent assaults in which the assaults are far worse than this. But the point in your case was the huge breach of trust which this constituted and the context in which you did it, as somebody in whom [Patient B] was placing natural and unthinking trust; and it was a very considerable ordeal for her when, over a period of some three quarters of an hour, you treated her in this sexualised and degrading way.'

The Panel found Patient A to be a reliable and credible witness. The Panel heard evidence from a close friend of Patient A and from her counsellor, both of whom told the Panel that they had been made aware of her relationship with Dr X. Although Patient A had already disclosed the matter to her counsellor and to her friend, she lodged a complaint against Dr X following the media publicity concerning the indecent assault on Patient B.

In the light of the allegations against Dr X concerning the indecent assault on Patient B, he was further requested by the Professional Sub Group of the Trust, in a letter from Dr E [date], only to consult with, and examine, unaccompanied female patients in the presence of a chaperone. Dr X agreed to comply with this. Whilst the Panel acknowledges that the whole issue of chaperoning was unclear within the practice, it considers that Dr X was an experienced practitioner and, as such, should have been acutely aware of what was required of him and what he had agreed to when undertaking consultations with female patients. The Panel does not accept that it was a matter for the practice staff to implement and maintain an effective system. It was Dr X's responsibility to take the necessary steps to ensure that the chaperoning requirements of the Trust were complied with, both in terms of the actual chaperone arrangements and in the monitoring thereof.

The Panel is concerned about the serious nature of the proven allegations against Dr X. Doctors occupy a position of privilege and trust in society and are expected to act with integrity and to uphold proper standards of conduct. The public has a right to expect that a doctor will behave in an appropriate and professional manner. Dr X's behaviour fell far short of these standards. In relation to Patient A it was compounded by the fact that he knew that she was vulnerable.

The Panel is in no doubt that Dr X's behaviour fell seriously below the standards expected of a registered medical practitioner.

In deciding whether Dr X's fitness to practise is impaired, the panel has had regard to the Indicative Sanctions Guidance when considering impaired fitness to practise. In particular page S1-2, paragraph 11, states: '…the GMC's role in relation to fitness to practise is to consider concerns which are so serious as to raise the question whether the doctor concerned should continue to practise either with restrictions on registration or at all'. Paragraph 58 on pages S3-14 and S3-15, states: 'A question of impaired fitness to practise is likely to arise if: A doctor has abused a patient's trust or violated a patient's autonomy or other fundamental rights: conduct which shows that a doctor has acted without regard for patients' rights or feelings, or has abused their professional position as a doctor, will usually give rise to questions about a doctor's fitness to practise'. The Panel considers that Dr X's behaviour has demonstrated that he cannot justify the trust placed in him. He has also, through this abuse of trust, undermined the confidence that members of the public place in the profession. Dr X has breached the fundamental principles of Good Medical Practice.

The conviction for indecent assault on Patient B, in itself, leads the Panel to conclude that Dr X's fitness to practise is impaired. The Panel has also determined that Dr X's inappropriate and improper behaviour with Patient A and also his failure to follow the recommendations of the Trust with regard to the chaperoning of unaccompanied female patients amounts to misconduct. The Panel therefore determines that Dr X's fitness to practise is impaired by reason of his misconduct and also by reason of his conviction for indecent assault on Patient B.

Case 5

Summary

The doctor had sexual intercourse with a vulnerable patient.

Relevant paragraphs of Good Medical Practice

The case relates to the *Relationships with patients* section of GMP, specifically paragraph 32 on maintaining trust in the profession. It also relates to the *Probity* section, specifically paragraph 57 on being honest and trustworthy.

Determination on impaired fitness to practise

Dr X is not present or represented at this hearing. The Panel has considered your submission that notification of this hearing has been properly served upon Dr X and that the Panel should proceed in his absence.

You have informed the Panel that the notice of this hearing, [date], was served on Dr X at his registered address. The Panel has noted the letter from [solicitor, date], confirming that Dr X is aware of these proceedings and that neither Dr X nor his legal representatives will be attending. The letter further stated that Dr X is content for the case to proceed in his absence.

The Panel has accepted that the General Medical Council has produced evidence, by way of the letter [date], which demonstrates that notification of today's proceedings has been properly served upon Dr X in accordance with Rule 40 of its Procedure Rules and paragraph 8(2)(d) of Schedule 4 of the Medical Act 1983 (as amended). In all the circumstances the Panel determined to proceed with the hearing in Dr X's absence, pursuant to Rule

31 of its Procedure Rules. The Panel has considered a letter from [solicitor, date] and notes that Dr X has admitted all of the allegations as set out in the Notice of Hearing [date]. The Panel has therefore recorded allegations 1–14 as admitted and found proved in their entirety.

The admissions are that: a) From around [date] Dr X, his wife and a third doctor were partners in general practice at the X Surgery, X. From around [date] to [date], Dr X and his wife used their family home ('X House') to provide residence for people with social and emotional problems. In a letter to the GMC dated [date], Dr X described this use of his family home as providing 'an extended family type of therapeutic community'. b) On or around [date], L and her young baby came to live with Dr X and his family at X House. L had been referred to Dr X by way of an emergency referral from Eating Disorders Support Service in X and/or [the Helpline]. L had a history of severe mental abuse, sexual abuse, physical abuse, psychological stress, satanic abuse and eating disorders. c) In [date], L's baby developed an acute abdominal complaint late one evening. Dr X arranged direct assessment for L's baby on the paediatric ward of X General Hospital. Dr X drove L and her baby to X General Hospital late that night. In relation to this incident Dr X acted in a professional capacity towards L and L's baby, as a general practitioner. d) On or around [date], L moved out of X House into temporary accommodation in X. In [date], L's mental state was deteriorating. On or around [date], Dr X prescribed to L 10 mg tablets of Amitriptyline and referred L to the Crisis Resolution Team of the community Health Team, X. The Crisis Resolution Team accepted the referral from Dr X as L's referring general practitioner and he did not inform the Team that this was not the case. By prescribing for L and referring her to the Crisis Resolution Team, Dr X acted in a professional capacity as her general practitioner. On [date] L was discharged from the Crisis Resolution Team. Dr X had a detailed knowledge of L's personal history, mental condition and degree of vulnerability. Dr X held a long term interest in mental health issues and had a lead role in strategic planning of mental health issues within the Primary Care Trust (PCT). On [date] and [date] Dr X went to L's temporary accommodation in X and engaged in sexual intercourse with her. L was classified as a vulnerable adult by mental health professionals.

Dr X has accepted that his actions were inappropriate, unprofessional, not in the best interests of L, an abuse of his position of trust as a registered medical practitioner and liable to bring the profession into disrepute.

The Panel has considered, on the basis of the allegations found proved, whether Dr X's fitness to practise is impaired by reason of his misconduct. In doing so, it has taken into account the written evidence before it, the oral evidence of Dr A, Consultant Psychiatrist, and the evidence of two Community Psychiatric Nurses. It has further noted that Dr X's solicitors, in their letter of [date], have confirmed that 'the existence of impairment by virtue of misconduct' is admitted. However, the question of his impairment is a matter for this Panel exercising its own professional judgement.

The Panel has had regard to the advice provided in the GMC's Indicative Sanctions Guidance. Paragraph 11 states that: 'Neither the Act nor the Rules define what is meant by impaired fitness to practise but for the reasons explained below, it is clear that the GMC's role in relation to fitness to practise is to consider concerns which are so serious as to raise the question whether the doctor concerned should continue to practise either with restrictions on registration or at all'. The Panel has considered Good Medical Practice (May 2001 edition) applicable at the time, which states that: 'You must not allow your personal relationships to undermine the trust which patients place in you. In particular, you must not use your professional position to establish or pursue a sexual or improper emotional relationship with a patient". It has also borne in mind the Indicative Sanctions Guidance Page S3-14 and S3-15, paragraph 58, which states that: 'A question of impaired fitness to practise is likely to arise if: … A doctor has abused a patient's trust or violated a patient's autonomy or other fundamental rights'.

The Panel has been informed that X House had a general policy to encourage residents to register with another practice in X to reduce the risk of any conflict of interest. However, some individuals were allowed to register with the practice if they wished. L was permitted to register with the X Surgery under the care of Dr B, Dr X's professional partner who worked part time in the practice. The Panel has heard that Dr X became closely involved with L's care and when he referred her to the Crisis Resolution Team they believed that he did so as her GP.

The Panel has not heard oral evidence from L at this hearing. However, it has heard from Dr A, Consultant Psychiatrist who became involved in L's care when Dr X referred her to the Crisis Resolution Team on [date]. Dr A told the Panel that she was concerned that L had been living at the home of Dr X and his wife and that despite her very significant history of severe mental illness, there had been no earlier involvement of the local mental health services in L's care. Dr A felt that Dr X had allowed a blurring of the professional and personal boundaries between L and himself. She told the Panel that she had assessed L as vulnerable and in need of community care: L had a poor ability to protect herself from sexual exploitation or significant harm from others, poor skills in assertiveness and had difficulty in saying 'no'. Nurse C confirmed that L was an extremely vulnerable patient.

Dr X was an experienced GP with a special interest in mental health issues and he was aware of L's mental health problems and extremely disturbed background, which involved sexual abuse. He was well placed to understand this vulnerability and indeed was sufficiently concerned about her health and wellbeing as to refer her to the Crisis Resolution Team on X.

Against this background, Dr X's behaviour in engaging in sexual intercourse with L on [date], soon after referring her to the Crisis Resolution Team, and subsequently pursuing this sexual relationship on [date] was wholly unprofessional. The Panel is greatly concerned at

Dr X's poor judgement and failure to maintain the proper professional boundaries by behaving in a way which he himself has acknowledged was: inappropriate, unprofessional, not in the best interests of L, an abuse of his position of trust as a registered medical practitioner, liable to bring the profession into disrepute.

The Panel has accordingly, pursuant to Section 35C(2)(a) of The Medical Act 1983 as amended, determined that Dr X's fitness to practise is impaired by reason of his misconduct.

Case 6

Summary

The doctor, having recently referred a female patient (a family friend) to the mental health team, visited her at home (after her father contacted him, concerned about her welfare) and engaged in sexual activity with her.

Relevant paragraphs of Good Medical Practice

The case relates to the *Relationships with patients* section of GMP, specifically paragraph 32 on maintaining trust in the profession, and paragraphs 21b and 21d on the doctor–patient partnership. It also relates to paragraph 57 of the *Probity* section on being honest and trustworthy.

Determination on impaired fitness to practise

Dr X is not present or represented at this hearing. The Panel has previously announced its findings on the facts. It has heard the submissions made by you and has considered the evidence of the witnesses called on behalf of the GMC. The Panel notes that Dr X gave no instructions to his solicitors in relation to any of the allegations. The Panel accepts the Legal Assessor's advice not to draw any inference from Dr X's decision not to participate in these proceedings.

The Panel found the following facts proved: At all material times Dr X was a General Practitioner principal practising from the X Medical Centre ('the practice'). At all material times Ms A was a registered patient at the practice and he was her General Practitioner. In [date] Dr X referred Ms A to the Mental Health Team because he was concerned about her general mental health.

In [date] Ms A's father contacted Dr X expressing concerns about his daughter's welfare. Dr X attended at Ms A's home where he let himself in with a key previously provided to him by Ms A. During the visit Dr X engaged in sexual activities with Ms A in her bed in that he put his hands inside Ms A's shorts and touched her under her clothing and put his hands on her breasts. Dr X remained in bed with Ms A until about 6:00 hours the following morning. On [date], Ms A made a complaint to Dr B. As a result of that complaint Dr X was contacted by Dr C. On [date], Dr C told Dr X not to discuss the matter with Ms A. Dr X subsequently contacted Ms A on her mobile telephone.

The Panel found that Dr X's actions were sexually motivated and were inappropriate, an abuse of his professional position and not in the best interests of Ms A. The Panel has considered, on the basis of the allegations found proved, whether Dr X's fitness to practise is impaired by reason of his misconduct. In doing so, it has taken into account the written evidence before it, in particular the witness statement of Ms A and the oral evidence of the witnesses called on behalf of the GMC.

The Panel has heard that at the relevant time, Ms A was a registered patient of Dr X. He was also a close family friend and their families had socialised together. Dr X was given a key to her front door so he could let himself in to take her dog out. Dr X knew of her personal problems and had referred her for counselling when she was suffering from depression in late [date]. In relation to the incident in question, Ms A states that in [date], Dr X telephoned her at home and asked her if she was OK as her father was concerned about her. She said she was OK and that she was going to bed. She acknowledged that she was on anti-depressants at the time and had consumed alcohol. She recalls that at some point she woke up and became aware that Dr X was present in the room. She realised that he must have used the key she had given to him to let himself into her home. He climbed into bed with her and started cuddling her. He got undressed, save for his t-shirt and boxer shorts. Dr X then proceeded to put his hands inside her shorts, touching her pubic area and made a comment that he thought she would have shaved. She responded 'well I don't' and he then put his hands on her breasts. She stated that she didn't know what to do about what was happening and 'brushed him off, moved away from him and curled up'. She stated that Dr X did not touch her again but stayed in bed with her until around 6am when he got up and left to go to work. She states that shortly after this incident, she had an appointment with Dr B, Psychiatrist who asked why she was upset and so told her of the incident with Dr X.

The Panel heard evidence from Dr B who confirmed that Ms A was seen in the outpatient clinic on [date] following an urgent referral by Dr X for a mental health assessment to be conducted. Dr B told the Panel that Ms A came with her parents who provided a history and were then asked to leave the room. Ms A then confided to her the incident with Dr X. Dr B stated that although she could smell alcohol on Ms A's breath, she did not appear to be intoxicated. Dr B concluded that Ms A was neither fantasising nor deluded.

Ms A did not want to make a formal complaint but was told that due to the nature of the allegation the matter would have to be referred to the PCT. Dr B's line manager contacted Ms E, Internal Governance Manager at the PCT. Ms A was called to a meeting with Ms E to give her version of the events and a statement was taken.

Ms E initiated an investigation into the complaint by asking Dr C, the then Chairman of the Professional Executive Committee to conduct a preliminary investigation. Dr C told the Panel that after speaking to Ms E on [date], he spoke to the psychiatric team who had seen Ms A and then telephoned Dr X. A meeting was arranged for the same day. Dr X told Dr C that he had cuddled Ms A on occasions but denied that any sexual activity had taken place between them. Dr C advised Dr X not to contact Ms A. However, he was told later that same day that Dr X had indeed contacted the patient.

Ms A in her statement also confirms that about a week after the incident, Dr X contacted her on her mobile. He told her that he was being accused of having sex with her, to which she replied that she had only told the truth and that he had upset her. He apologised to her but she said it was too late as he had 'destroyed her trust'.

The Panel also heard the evidence of Dr D, Dr X's partner at the practice. Dr D told the Panel that he saw Ms A in consultation on [dates] and that at both these consultations Ms A informed him of the incident in question. Dr D stated that Ms A had not wanted to make a formal complaint against Dr X. Dr D stated that as he felt out of his depth he contacted the MDU for advice. He also contacted Dr B and the PCT and spoke to Dr C who told him that Dr X had been told to explain the events to him. A practice meeting was then held where Dr X admitted going to Ms A's house, kissing and cuddling her and staying the night. Dr X told him that allegations made against him were investigated by the PCT which had concluded the matter. Dr D told the Panel that he had, previous to this incident, provided 25 per cent of Ms A's care but since then was now 100 per cent responsible for her care.

Following Dr C's preliminary investigation, an oral hearing was held on [date] at the PCT, the purpose of which was to consider Dr X's continued inclusion on the PCT's Performer's List. Ms E gave evidence that during the PCT hearing, Dr X's explanation for his conduct was that after receiving a telephone call from Ms A's father expressing his concerns regarding her excessive drinking, he rang Ms A who agreed that it was OK for him to visit her at home. He went on to state that when he arrived at Ms A's house she suggested opening a bottle of wine, which he declined as he was driving. He claims that Ms A then said to him 'I'm going to bed now are you coming?' Dr X stated that he slipped into his underpants and they cuddled and kissed. He admitted putting his hand under her top and feeling her breasts and putting his hand inside her pyjama bottoms over her mons pubis area. He then said to her 'you trust me completely don't you', to which she replied 'yes or uh huh' at which point he removed his hand and they went to sleep.

As stated in the Panel's determination on the facts the Panel found the evidence of Ms A to be consistent with the live witnesses as opposed to Dr X's accounts to Dr C and Dr D and to the oral hearing which were not consistent. The Panel has considered, on the basis of the allegations found proved, whether Dr X's fitness to practise is impaired by reason of his misconduct bearing in mind that the question of Dr X's impairment is a matter for this Panel exercising its own professional judgement.

The Panel has had regard to the advice provided in the GMC's Indicative Sanctions Guidance. Paragraph 11 states that: 'Neither the Act nor the Rules define what is meant by impaired fitness to practise but for the reasons explained below, it is clear that the GMC's role in relation to fitness to practise is to consider concerns which are so serious as to raise the question whether the doctor concerned should continue to practise either with restrictions on registration or at all'.

The Panel has considered Good Medical Practice (May 2001 edition) applicable at the time, which states that: 'You must not allow your personal relationships to undermine the trust which patients place in you. In particular, you must not use your professional position to establish or pursue a sexual or improper emotional relationship with a patient'. It has also borne in mind the Indicative Sanctions Guidance and in particular, paragraph 54 states: '… Doctors have a respected position in society and their work gives them privileged access to patients, some of whom may be very vulnerable. A doctor whose conduct has shown that he cannot justify the trust placed in him should not continue in unrestricted practice while that remains the case'. And Paragraph 58, which states that: 'A question of impaired fitness to practise is likely to arise if: A doctor has abused a patient's trust or violated a patient's autonomy or other fundamental rights'.

The Panel has been informed that Dr X is an experienced GP and as well as being Ms A's GP for a period of 20 years, was also a close family friend. He was aware of Ms A's fragile state of health and was well placed to understand this vulnerability. Indeed he was sufficiently concerned about her health and wellbeing to refer her for counselling in late [date] and to make an urgent telephone referral to the Mental Health Team in [date]. Against this background, Dr X's behaviour, in engaging in sexual activity with Ms A in [date] and subsequently telephoning her after he was told that a complaint had been made, was wholly unprofessional. Although the Panel acknowledges that this was a single isolated incident of misconduct, it was a very serious breach of Ms A's trust. The Panel is greatly concerned at Dr X's poor judgement and failure to maintain the proper professional boundaries by behaving in a way which the Panel has found to be inappropriate, an abuse of his position of trust as a registered medical practitioner and not in the best interests of Ms A.

The Panel has accordingly, pursuant to Section 35C(2)(a) of The Medical Act 1983 as amended, determined that Dr X's fitness to practise is impaired by reason of his misconduct.

Case 7

Summary

The doctor gave his personal mobile number to a patient who he examined at A&E and pursued a sexual relationship with her at the same time as acting – or purporting to act – as her doctor. He signed a letter as her doctor stating that he was Acting Consultant Emergency Medicine when this was not the case.

Relevant paragraphs of Good Medical Practice

The case relates to the *Relationships with patients* section of GMP, specifically paragraph 32 on maintaining trust in the profession. It also relates to the *Probity* section, specifically paragraphs 63 and 65 on signing documents.

Determination on impaired fitness to practise

Pursuant to Rule 17(2)(k), the Panel has considered, on the basis of the facts it found proved in [date], whether Dr X's fitness to practise is impaired. In doing so it has considered all the evidence adduced and your submissions on behalf of the General Medical Council (GMC).

The GMC's Indicative Sanctions Guidance states at page S3-13, paragraphs 54 and 55, that: 'Doctors have a respected position in society and their work gives them privileged access to patients, some of whom may be very vulnerable. A doctor whose conduct has shown that he cannot justify the trust placed in him should not continue in unrestricted practice while that remains the case. In short, the public is entitled to expect that their doctor is fit to practise, and follows the GMC's principles of good practice described in Good Medical Practice'.

The Panel has found Dr X's actions to be inappropriate, an abuse of his position as a registered medical practitioner, below the standard expected of a medical practitioner, and dishonest.

Dr X first examined Miss A at the Accident & Emergency Department of X Hospital on [date]. At Dr X's request Miss A returned to the Accident & Emergency Department on [dates]. During the consultation on [date], Dr X gave Miss A his personal mobile telephone number. Miss A texted Dr X and he responded on matters unconnected with her medical condition, with text messages which were flirtatious in manner. When Miss A returned to the Accident & Emergency Department on [date], Dr X engaged in flirtatious conversation with her during the examination of her injured knee. The Panel found that Dr X's actions in giving Miss A his personal mobile number, responding to her text messages on matters unconnected with her medical condition, and engaging in flirtatious text messaging and conversation with her, whilst being a medical practitioner responsible for her clinical care, were inappropriate and an abuse of his position as a registered medical practitioner.

In [dates] Dr X suggested he and Miss A meet up on several occasions. From [date] to around [date – 11 months later] Dr X pursued a sexual relationship with Miss A and was also sexually intimate with her whilst on duty at the Accident & Emergency Department, which the Panel found to be inappropriate and an abuse of his position as a registered medical practitioner.

During the course of their sexual relationship Dr X acted or purported to act in a professional capacity in relation to Miss A. On [date] he signed a Statutory Sick Pay Form for Miss A, as her doctor at X General Hospital. He also provided Miss A with a letter dated [date], as her doctor, confirming that she was fit to return to work. In that letter he also stated that he was 'Acting Consultant Emergency Medicine'. The Panel found Dr X's actions in these instances to be inappropriate, below the standard expected of a medical practitioner, and dishonest. Dr X was not Miss A's doctor at those times and was not, nor had he ever been, 'Acting Consultant Emergency Medicine'.

The Panel is aware of its responsibility to protect the public interest, with particular reference to maintaining public confidence in the profession and upholding proper standards of conduct and behaviour. The public are entitled to expect that doctors will be honest and trustworthy at all times.

The GMC's Good Medical Practice 2001 states at paragraph 20 that: 'You must not allow your personal relationships to undermine the trust which patients place in you. In particular, you must not use your professional position to establish or pursue a sexual or improper emotional relationship with a patient or someone close to them' and at paragraph 51 that: 'You must be honest and trustworthy when writing reports, completing or signing forms. ... You must not write or sign documents which are false...'. The Panel has determined that Dr X's actions fell seriously short of the standards of behaviour the public are entitled to expect from doctors and undermines public confidence in the profession.

In the circumstances, the Panel has determined that Dr X's fitness to practise is impaired by reason of his misconduct, pursuant to Section 35C(2)(a) of the Medical Act 1983 (as amended).

Case 8

Summary

The doctor carried out inappropriate intimate examinations on a female patient and did not make a note of the examinations in the patient's medical record.

Relevant paragraphs of Good Medical Practice

The case relates to the *Probity* section of GMP, specifically paragraph 57 on being honest and trustworthy. It also relates to the *Relationships with patients* section, specifically paragraphs 21b and 21d on the doctor–patient partnership, and paragraph 32 on maintaining trust in the profession. Finally it relates to paragraphs 3f and 3g of the *Good clinical care* section on record-keeping.

Determination on impaired fitness to practise

At the material time you were a General Practitioner and partner at the X Surgery, X, (The Surgery). Patient A was a registered patient at that Surgery. On [date removed] you saw Patient A, who attended the surgery to consult you about dizziness and an ear infection. At that consultation, Patient A told you that following the removal of her contraceptive coil she had been experiencing heavy bleeding. You provided her with forms to undergo blood tests at X General Hospital. You asked her if you could undertake an internal examination but she declined the offer as she had her period at the time. The Panel has found that your request to undertake an internal examination on that occasion was inappropriate and not clinically justified.

On [date], Patient A consulted you again in order to get the results of the blood test. You discussed her ear infection and dizziness and the results of her blood test. You asked her about her periods, if she was sexually active and if she had a partner.

The Panel has heard that at that consultation you also commented on Patient A's attractiveness. This comment was inappropriate, improper, and liable to bring the profession into disrepute. You also asked her if you could carry out an internal examination. The Panel has found this request was not clinically justified. Patient A reluctantly agreed to an internal examination. You did not explain why it was necessary to conduct an internal examination nor what the clinical benefit would be. You neither offered her the presence of a chaperone, friend or relative, nor did you afford her appropriate privacy during the examination which followed. Your actions and omissions were inappropriate, improper and not in the best interests of the patient.

Once Patient A was undressed, you asked her about her naval piercing, began to fiddle with the piercing with your fingers and bent down and examined it through your cupped hands. The Panel has found this behaviour to have been inappropriate, an abuse of your position of trust, not in the best interests of the patient and indecent.

The Panel has found that you then purported to conduct an internal examination by inserting your fingers into Patient A's vagina and sliding your fingers in and out on a number of occasions. This was neither a proper internal examination, nor was it was clinically justified. Further, it was inappropriate, indecent and not in the best interests of the patient. It was an abuse of your position of trust and liable to bring the profession into disrepute.

Following the internal examination, you asked Patient A about her breasts. She informed you that she had had breast surgery about four months previously. At your request, she exposed her breasts and then you cupped your hand around her right breast and tweaked her right nipple. Your actions were not clinically justified, not a proper breast examination, inappropriate, indecent, not in the best interests of the patient, an abuse of your position of trust and liable to bring the profession into disrepute.

Following the examination, you told Patient A that you would telephone her on the following Monday to make sure she was all right. You commented on a previous experience which you had had with an elderly patient asking for internal examinations. Your remarks were inappropriate. Further, you did not record in her medical notes that you had purported to conduct internal and breast examinations. Your failure to make a record of your examinations was inappropriate.

The GMC publication 'Good Medical Practice' (2001) states clearly that 'patients must be able to trust doctors with their lives and well-being. To justify that trust, we as a profession have a duty to maintain a good standard of practice and care and to show respect for human life. In particular as a doctor you must: Treat every patient politely and considerately; Respect patients' dignity and privacy; Be honest and trustworthy; Avoid abusing your position as a doctor'. It further states that 'Successful relationships between doctors and patients depend on trust'. Additionally: 'In providing care you must keep clear, accurate, legible and contemporaneous patient records which report the relevant clinical findings, the decisions made, the information given to patients and any drugs or other treatment prescribed'. You failed to adhere to these requirements.

Your actions and conduct in relation to this patient, constitute fundamental breaches of the principles and standards expected of a registered doctor and represent a gross abuse of the doctor/patient relationship. Accordingly, the Panel has found that your fitness to practise is impaired because of your misconduct.

Website resources and information

Royal College of Psychiatrists

Web pages

Psychiatrists' Support Service
http://www.rcpsych.ac.uk/member/psychiatristssupportservice.aspx

CPD Online
http://www.rcpsych.ac.uk/publications/cpdonline.aspx

Resource Catalogue
http://www.rcpsych.ac.uk/mentalhealthinfoforall/moreinformation/
ordermaterials.aspx

Documents

Good Psychiatric Practice (3rd edition) (Council Report CR154), 2009. http://
www.rcpsych.ac.uk/publications/collegereports/cr/cr154.aspx

Vulnerable Patients, Vulnerable Doctors. Good Practice in Our Clinical Relationships
(Council Report CR146), 2007. http://www.rcpsych.ac.uk/publications/
collegereports/cr/cr146.aspx

Sexual Boundary Issues in Psychiatric Settings (Council Report CR 145). http://
www.rcpsych.ac.uk/publications/collegereports/cr/cr145.aspx

Major inquiries

Ayling Inquiry report, 2004
http://www.dh.gov.uk/en/Publicationsandstatistics/Publications/
PublicationsPolicyAndGuidance/DH_4088996

Independent Investigation into the Conduct of David Britten, 2008
http://www.verita.net/pages/our_work/107/verita.html

The Kerr/Haslam Inquiry, 2005
http://www.dh.gov.uk/en/Publicationsandstatistics/Publications/
PublicationsPolicyAndGuidance/DH_4115349

The Neale Inquiry, 2004
http://www.dh.gov.uk/en/Publicationsandstatistics/Publications/
PublicationsPolicyAndGuidance/DH_4088995

The Ritchie report, 2000 (concerning Rodney Ledward)
http://www.dh.gov.uk/en/Publicationsandstatistics/Publications/
PublicationsPolicyAndGuidance/DH_4093337

The Shipman Inquiry, 2002
http://www.the-shipman-inquiry.org.uk/reports.asp

Council for Healthcare Regulatory Excellence (CRHE)

http://www.chre.org.uk

Reports from the CHRE

Clear Sexual Boundaries
http://www.chre.org.uk/satellite/133

Gives access to:
- *Guidance for Patients on Clear Sexual Boundaries With Healthcare Professionals*
- *Clear Sexual Boundaries Between Healthcare Professionals and Patients: Responsibilities of Healthcare Professionals*
- *Clear Sexual Boundaries Between Healthcare Professionals and Patients: Guidance for Fitness to Practise Panels*
- *Learning About Sexual Boundaries Between Healthcare Professionals and Patients: A Report on Education and Training*
- *Sexual Boundary Violations by Health Professionals – An Overview of the Published Empirical Literature*

Other organisations

Clinic for Boundary Studies (formerly Witness)
http://professionalboundaries.org.uk

General Medical Council (GMC)
http://www.gmc-uk.org

National Patient Safety Agency (NPSA)
http://www.npsa.nhs.uk

Public Concern at Work (PCAW)
http://www.pcaw.co.uk

Index

Compiled by Linda English

RCPsych Publications is the publishing imprint of the Royal College of Psychiatrists. We have also published the following titles you may be interested in:

Social Inclusion and Mental Health

Edited by Jed Boardman, Alan Currie, Helen Killaspy and Gillian Mezey

Gives advice on facilitating the social inclusion of people with mental health problems.

ISBN: 978-1-904671-87-9, price £30

Nidotherapy: Harmonising the Environment with the Patient

By Peter Tyrer

An introductory guide to the emerging treatment of nidotherapy.

ISBN: 978-1-904671-74-9, price £10

Primary Care Mental Health

Edited by Linda Gask, Helen Lester, Tony Kendrick and Robert Peveler

Practical advice about how practitioners in primary care can best respond to psychiatric presentations.

ISBN: 978-1-904671-77-0, price £35

Winner of the
BMA Medical Book Award 2010
(Primary health care category)

Emergency Department Handbook: Children and Adolescents with Mental Health Problems

Edited by Tony Kaplan

A practical handbook covering everything a practitioner needs to know about dealing with young people who present in an emergency department with mental health problems.

ISBN: 978-1-904671-73-2, price £15

The Mind: A User's Guide

Consultant Editor: Raj Persaud

An accessible, jargon-free book for anyone who has an interest in safeguarding or improving their mental health.

ISBN: 978-0-593056-35-6, price £14.99

The Young Mind

Co-edited by Sue Bailey and Mike Shooter

This is an accessible, user-friendly handbook for parents, teachers and young adults.

ISBN: 978-0-593061-38-1, price £14.99

Mental Health Outcome Measures (3rd edn)

Edited by Graham Thornicroft and Michele Tansella

A guide to the minefield area of outcome measurement.

ISBN: 978-1-904671-92-3, price £30

Clinical Topics in Cultural Psychiatry

Edited by Rahul Bhattacharya, Sean Cross and Dinesh Bhugra

Practical advice about the way psychiatric symptoms are presented to clinicians and how clinicians should deal with them.

ISBN: 978-1-904671-82-4, price £30

Fish's Clinical Psychopathology: Signs and Symptoms in Psychiatry (3rd edn)

By Patricia Casey and Brendan Kelly

This classic text presents the clinical descriptions and psychopathological insights of Fish to a new generation.

ISBN: 978-1-904671-32-9, price £18

Please contact Book Sales at the Royal College of Psychiatrists, +44 (0)20 7235 2351 x6146, or order online at:
www.rcpsych.ac.uk/publications
Our trade distributors (UK) are Turpin distribution.
We also have distributors in the USA and Australia.

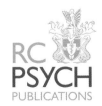

RC
PSYCH
PUBLICATIONS

The Royal College of Psychiatrists

CPD ONLINE

Interactive learning for mental health professionals

The CPD Online website provides learning modules using a range of multimedia techniques. It is relevant for fully qualified psychiatrists and other mental health professionals and can be used to acquire up to 10 external hours of core learning towards your continuing professional development (CPD) requirements.

Learning modules are all peer-reviewed and provide a dynamic and rich information source to improve your knowledge, help you to acquire new skills quickly, and enable you to keep up to date with new research and best practice in psychiatry.

There are currently over 97 modules to choose from, with more being developed all the time. There are also 51 modules based on podcasts of interviews with leading psychiatrists, specially produced for CPD Online.

Most modules take between 30 minutes and an hour to finish and on successful completion of the module you can print out a certificate for your records. There is a personalised 'My CPD' area that records module progress and stores certificates gained. Try out our free sample modules via a guest account.

www.psychiatrycpd.org

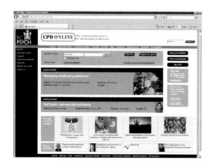

Primary Care Mental Health

**Winner of the
BMA Medical Book
Award 2010**
(Primary health care
category)

**Edited by Linda Gask, Helen Lester,
Tony Kendrick and Robert Peveler**

Primary care is usually the first port of call for
people with mental health problems and plays an
increasingly important role in developing and delivering
mental health services. Indeed, 90% of all patients with mental health
problems (including 30–50% of all those with serious mental illness) only
use primary care services.

How can practitioners in primary care best respond to psychiatric
presentations? In this book, internationally respected authors provide a
conceptual background and dispense practical advice for the clinician.
They discuss ways of improving joint working between primary and
secondary care, as well as issues affecting the professional development of
all practitioners within primary care teams.

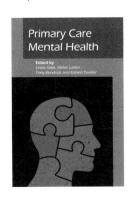

Key features include:

- Practical advice
- Focus on improving services
- Educational strategies to develop knowledge and
  skills of the primary care team
- Critical analysis of the emerging evidence
- A user-centred approach, emphasising recovery.

2009, hardback, 512 pages, ISBN: 978-1-904671-77-0, price £35.00
(RCPsych members' price: £31.50)

Please contact: Book Sales, Royal College of Psychiatrists,
17 Belgrave Square, London SW1X 8PG, UK.
Tel: +44 (0)20 7235 2351 ext 6146. Fax: +44 (0)20 7245 1231.
Order online: **www.rcpsych.ac.uk/publications**

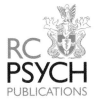

RC
PSYCH
PUBLICATIONS

Good Psychiatric Practice

Good Psychiatric Practice

Royal College of Psychiatrists

College Report CR154

Vulnerable patients, safe doctors

Good practice
in our clinical relationships

Royal College of Psychiatrists

College Report CR146

Good Psychiatric Practice

Relationships with
pharmaceutical and other
commercial organisations

Royal College of Psychiatrists

College Report CR148

Good Psychiatric Practice

Continuing professional
development

Royal College of Psychiatrists

College Report CR157

Good Psychiatric Practice: Confidentiality and Information Sharing

Royal College of Psychiatrists

College Report CR160

Royal College of Psychiatrists core guidance
for its members.

The Good Psychiatric Practice group of
documents is available freely at:
www.rcpsych.ac.uk/gpp

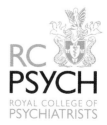

RC
PSYCH
ROYAL COLLEGE OF
PSYCHIATRISTS